P CKET
PIMPED
ORTHOPEDIC SURGERY

David B. Johnson, Jr.
Jacob J. Triplet

© 2019 Pocket Pimped, LLC
www.PocketPimped.com
ISBN: 978-0-578-43913-6

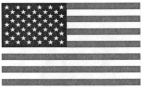

Printed in the United States of America

All rights reserved. No part of this book may be reproduced in any form, electronic or mechanical, for any reason or means, including photocopying. It may not be utilized by any information storage and retrieval system without written permission from the authors and owners.

NOTICE

Readers are to be advised that this book is not intended to guide medical or surgical decision making. Pocket Pimped, LLC, and its affiliated contributors, are not responsible for errors or omissions that may be present in this book. Moreover, they are not responsible for the consequences from application of the information contained within this book. The authors make no assurance, written or implied, that the contents of the book are accurate. Application of the information contained within this book remains the responsibility of the practitioner. Additionally, with continued research and regulation changes, the authors encourage the reader to refer to the most current literature. Again, it is the responsibility of the practitioner to make the diagnosis, and provide the best treatment for each individual patient. To the fullest extent of the law, neither the publisher nor the authors assume any liability for any damage and/or injury to property or persons related to any use of the material contained within this book.

Editors and Contributors

Benjamin C. Taylor, MD, FAAOS
Orthopedic Trauma Surgery
Fellowship Director, Grant Medical Center
Site Director, OTA International Traveling Fellowship
Site Director, AO Trauma Traveling Fellowship
Clinical Assistant Professor of Orthopedics, Ohio University
Assistant Program Director, OhioHealth Orthopedics
Editor-In-Chief, Orthobullets.com
Orthopedic Trauma and Reconstructive Surgeons
Columbus, OH

Jonathan C. Levy, MD, FAAOS
Shoulder and Elbow Surgery
Chief of Orthopedics, Holy Cross Hospital
Fellowship Director, Holy Cross Shoulder and Elbow Surgery
Medical Director, Holy Cross Orthopedic Research Institute
Holy Cross Medical Group
Fort Lauderdale, FL

Kevin E. Klingele, MD
Pediatric Orthopedic Surgery
Chief of Orthopedic Surgery, Nationwide Children's Hospital
Fellowship Director, Nationwide Children's Hospital
Director of Sports Medicine, Nationwide Children's Hospital
Adjunct Assistant Professor, The Ohio State University
Nationwide Children's Hospital
Columbus, OH

Editors and Contributors

Christopher A. Iobst, MD
Pediatric Orthopedic Surgery
Fellowship Director, Limb Lengthening and Reconstruction
Director, Center for Limb Lengthening and Reconstruction
Clinical Associate Professor, The Ohio State University
Nationwide Children's Hospital
Columbus, OH

Terrance M. Philbin, DO
Foot and Ankle Surgery
Fellowship Director, Orthopedic Foot and Ankle Center
Orthopedic Foot and Ankle Center
Westerville, OH

Quincy P. Samora III, MD
Pediatric Orthopedic Surgery
Residency Director, Nationwide Children's Hospital
Clinical Assistant Professor, The Ohio State University
Nationwide Children's Hospital
Columbus, OH

Julie B. Samora, MD, PhD
Pediatric Hand and Upper Extremity Surgery
Director, Hand and Upper Extremity Research
Director, Orthopedic Quality Improvement
Clinical Associate Professor, The Ohio State University
Nationwide Children's Hospital
Columbus, OH

Editors and Contributors

Ray C. Wasielewski, MD
Adult Reconstruction Surgery
Medical Director, OhioHealth Bone & Joint Center
OhioHealth Orthopedic Surgeons
Grant Medical Center
Columbus, OH

Nathan G. Everding, MD
Shoulder, Elbow and Hand Surgery
Syracuse Orthopedic Specialists
Syracuse, NY

B. Rodney Comisar, MD
Sports Medicine Surgery
Team Physician, Denison University
Chairman, Clinical Guidance Council Grant Medical Center
OrthoNeuro
Columbus, OH

F. Paul DeGenova, DO
Orthopedic Spine Surgeon
Chairman, Department of Orthopedics Grant Medical Center
OhioHealth Orthopedic Surgeons
Grant Medical Center
Columbus, OH

David K. Galos, MD
Orthopedic Trauma Surgery
Assistant Professor of Orthopedic Surgery, Hofstra University
Northwell Health
Garden City, NY

To our wives and children, whose continued love,
support, and understanding made this book possible.

Contents

The Basics   1

I. X-rays 2
- Upper Extremity
- Pelvis
- Lower Extremity

II. Infections 8

III. Compartment Syndrome 12

IV. General Knowledge 16
- AO/OTA Classification
- Nonunions
- Closed Fractures
- Open Fractures
- Osteoporosis
- Cartilage
- Bone Formation
- Principles & Properties

Shoulder Girdle   25

I. General Anatomy 26

II. Trauma 32
- Clavicle
- Acromioclavicular (AC) Joint
- Scapula
- Proximal Humerus
- Shoulder Dislocations

III. Sports ... 38
- Rotator Cuff
- Shoulder Instability & Labrum
- Proximal Biceps
- Adhesive Capsulitis & GIRD

IV. Adult Reconstruction ... 45
- Shoulder Hemiarthroplasty
- Total Shoulder Arthroplasty (TSA)
- Reverse Shoulder Arthroplasty (RSA)

Arm   49
I. General Anatomy ... 50
II. Trauma ... 52
- Humerus

Elbow   55
I. General Anatomy ... 56
II. Trauma ... 61
- Capitellum & Trochlea
- Proximal Ulna
- Proximal Radius

III. Sports ... 64
- Elbow Instability
- Epicondylitis
- Distal Biceps

Forearm & Wrist   67
I. General Anatomy ... 68

II. Trauma 72
- Forearm
- Wrist

Hand — 77
I. General Anatomy 78
II. Hand Conditions 85
- Carpal Tunnel Syndrome
- Scaphoid
- Lunate
- Metacarpal
- Thumb
- Phalanx
- Trigger Finger
- Flexor Tendon Injuries
- Extensor Tendon Injuries
- Carpometacarpal Arthritis

Spine — 97
I. General Anatomy 98
II. Trauma 102
- Vertebral Fractures
- Spinal Cord Injuries

III. Spinal Conditions 105
- Cervical Myelopathy
- Ankylosing Spondylitis (AS)
- Diffuse Idiopathic Skeletal Hyperostosis

Pelvis — 107

- I. General Anatomy — 108
- II. Trauma — 110
  - Pelvic Ring

Hip — 113

- I. General Anatomy — 114
- II. Trauma — 117
  - Acetabulum
  - Hip Dislocations
  - Femoral Head & Neck
  - Intertrochanteric Fractures
  - Subtrochanteric Fractures
- III. Sports — 125
  - Femoracetabular Impingement (FAI)
  - Coxa Sultans (Snapping Hip)
- IV. Adult Reconstruction — 127
  - Total Hip Arthroplasty (THA)

Femur — 133

- I. General Anatomy — 134
- II. Trauma — 135
  - Femoral Shaft
  - Distal Femur

Knee — 139

- I. General Anatomy — 140

II. Trauma 145
- Patella
- Knee Dislocations
- Tibial Plateau

III. Sports 150
- Anterior Cruciate Ligament (ACL)
- Collateral Ligaments (MCL, LCL)
- Meniscus Injuries
- Discoid Meniscus
- Patella

IV. Adult Reconstruction 160
- Total Knee Arthroplasty (TKA)
- Unicompartmental Knee Arthroplasty (UKA)

Leg   167

I. General Anatomy 168
II. Trauma 170
- Tibial Shaft

Foot & Ankle   173

I. General Anatomy 174
II. Trauma 181
- Pilon
- Ankle
- Talus
- Subtalar Dislocations
- Calcaneus
- Lisfranc
- 5th Metatarsal

III. Foot & Ankle Conditions ... 192
- Achilles Tendon
- Peroneal Tendons
- Posterior Tibial Tendon Insufficiency (PTTI)
- Hallux Valgus
- Hallux Rigidus
- Cavovarus Foot
- Freiberg's Disease
- Lesser Toes

Pediatrics   201
I. General Anatomy ... 202
II. The Basics ... 206
- Physis
- Joint Hypermobility
- Lower Extremity Alignment
- Cerebral Palsy (CP)

III. Upper Extremity ... 211
- Little Leaguer's Shoulder
- Supracondylar Humerus
- Elbow
- Forearm & Wrist
- Hand
- Upper Extremity Syndromes & Conditions

IV. Spine ... 220
- Scoliosis
- Kyphosis
- Spondylolysis/Spondylolisthesis

V. Lower Extremity 225
- Developmental Dysplasia of the Hip (DDH)
- Legg-Calve-Perthes
- Slipped Capital Femoral Epiphysis (SCFE)
- Transient Synovitis vs Septic Arthritis
- Femur
- Leg Length Discrepancy (LLD)
- Blount's Disease
- Tibia
- Ankle
- Foot

Preface

The concept of pimping, or asking questions to test one's knowledge, is a longstanding tradition that provides perspective to an individual's preparedness and understanding of a topic. In orthopedic surgery, each operative case or disease process has a group of questions that are predictably asked. It was the recognition of this pattern that sparked the beginning of *Pocket Pimped*. This book is a collection of common pimp questions that we, as residents, fellows, and attendings either ask or have been asked. We hope that the reader may use this book as a resource to be better prepared and to guide their studies as they begin to decipher what is important in their journey to becoming an orthopedic surgeon. The authors wish the readers all the best in their pursuit.

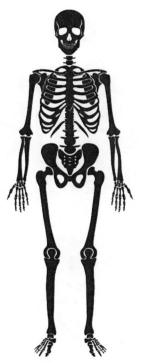

THE BASICS

The Basics

X-Rays

Upper Extremity

1. What view must always be obtained when evaluating a patient with a shoulder dislocation?
    ➢ Axillary
2. If an axillary view is not tolerated, what alternative view may be obtained?
    ➢ Velpeau
3. What radiographic finding is suggestive of a posterior shoulder dislocation?
    ➢ Light bulb sign
4. What view is a true AP of the glenohumeral joint?
    ➢ Grashey
5. The acromioclavicular (AC) joint is best visualized on what view?
    ➢ Zanca
6. The sternoclavicular (SC) joint is best visualized on what view?
    ➢ Serendipity
7. A Hill-Sachs lesion is best visualized on what view?
    ➢ Stryker Notch
8. A bony Bankart is best visualized on what view?
    ➢ West Point
9. What x-ray should be obtained to better evaluate intraarticular distal humerus fractures?
    ➢ Traction view
10. What radiographic finding suggests an occult fracture about the elbow?

- Posterior fat pad sign

11. Does an anterior fat pad sign suggest a fracture?
    - Not always, this can be a normal finding if the elbow is flexed
12. What radiographic finding indicates a capitellum fracture that extends to the trochlea?
    - Double-arc sign
13. What view of the wrist evaluates dorsal screw lengths following ORIF of the distal radius?
    - Skyline
14. How do you obtain a scaphoid view?
    - PA x-ray with maximal ulnar deviation
15. What are Gilula's arcs on a hand x-ray?
    - First arc: Proximal convexity of the scaphoid, lunate, and triquetrum
    - Second arc: Distal concavity of the scaphoid, lunate, and triquetrum
    - Third arc: Proximal convexity of the capitate and hamate

Pelvis

16. What are the 6 radiographic lines of the pelvis and what anatomic structures do they represent?
    - Iliopectineal line – Anterior column
    - Ilioischial line – Posterior column
    - Anterior wall
    - Posterior wall
    - Acetabular dome (Sourcil)
        - Sourcil is eyebrow in French
    - Tear drop – Medial acetabular wall

The Basics

17. What radiographs should be obtained to evaluate the pelvic ring?
    ➢ AP pelvis, inlet, and outlet views
18. What makes a perfect AP pelvis radiograph?
    ➢ Symmetric obturator foramen, midline spinous processes, coccyx is 2cm superior to the pubic ramus
19. What makes a perfect inlet radiograph?
    ➢ S1 overlying S2
20. What makes a perfect outlet radiograph?
    ➢ Pubic ramus overlying S2
21. The inlet view evaluates for displacement in which planes?
    ➢ AP and rotation
22. The outlet view evaluates for displacement in which planes?
    ➢ Superior-Inferior and Flexion-Extension
23. What series of radiographs should be obtained to evaluate the acetabulum?
    ➢ Judet views – Obturator oblique and Iliac oblique
24. The iliac oblique view evaluates which structures?
    ➢ Anterior wall and posterior column
        • Remember: **IOWA** (**I**liac **O**blique, **W**all **A**nterior)
25. The obturator oblique view evaluates which structures?
    ➢ Posterior wall and anterior column
26. What is Shenton's line?

The Basics

- ➢ Congruent line from the medial femoral neck extending to the superior portion of the obturator foramen

27. What is the "spur sign"?
    - ➢ Radiographic finding seen on the obturator oblique view that is pathognomonic for a both column acetabular fracture
        - ▪ The "spur" is the edge of the intact ilium

28. What is the "gull sign"?
    - ➢ Radiographic view of the fractured posterior wall that resembles a flying seagull
    - ➢ Can also be used to describe superomedial dome impaction seen in elderly patients

29. What is a positive "Throckmorton sign"?
    - ➢ Radiographic shadow of the penis points towards the side of the fracture

Lower Extremity

30. What radiograph should be obtained to better delineate the fracture pattern in intertrochanteric femur fractures?
    - ➢ Traction view

31. What additional radiograph must be obtained preoperatively for intertrochanteric femur fractures?
    - ➢ Full length femur x-ray to evaluate for distal hardware that may prevent passage of a nail

32. What is the difference between a cross table lateral and a frog leg lateral?
    - ➢ Frog leg: Lateral of the femur, AP of the pelvis
    - ➢ Cross table: Lateral of femur, lateral of the pelvis

The Basics

33. What position should the leg be placed in to obtain a true AP of the femur?
    ➢ 15° internal rotation to account for femoral anteversion
34. The cross-over sign on an AP pelvis x-ray is indicative of what condition?
    ➢ Pincer type femoroacetabular impingement
35. A pistol-grip deformity on a hip radiograph is indicative of what condition?
    ➢ Cam type femoroacetabular impingement
36. What makes a perfect AP radiograph of the knee?
    ➢ Fibula is bisected by the lateral aspect of the proximal tibia
37. What makes a perfect lateral radiograph of the knee?
    ➢ The medial and lateral femoral condyles are superimposed
38. Which radiographic view of the knee typically shows the earliest evidence of arthritis?
    ➢ Rosenberg
39. What three radiographic views of the ankle should always be obtained?
    ➢ AP, lateral and mortise
40. What makes a perfect lateral x-ray of the ankle?
    ➢ The talar domes are superimposed
41. How is a mortise view obtained?
    ➢ Internal rotation of the leg 15°
42. What are the radiographic lines of the foot on AP, oblique and lateral x-rays?

> AP: Medial border of the 2nd metatarsal should line up with the medial border of the middle cuneiform
> Oblique: Medial aspect of the 4th metatarsal should line up with the medial aspect of the cuboid
> Lateral: Proximal aspect of the metatarsals should not be dorsally displaced relative to cuneiforms

43. What view is best for visualizing the talar neck?
> Canale

44. What two specific radiographs should be obtained to evaluate the calcaneus?
> Harris and Broden views

The Basics
Infections

45. What three laboratory tests should be obtained in all patients being worked up for infection?
    - ➤ ESR, CRP, WBC
46. What laboratory value is trended to monitor for improvement in acute infections?
    - ➤ CRP
47. Which laboratory tests should be ordered on synovial fluid samples?
    - ➤ Gram stain
    - ➤ Synovial fluid analysis – includes WBC
    - ➤ Cultures – aerobic, anaerobic, fungus, acid-fast
    - ➤ Protein and glucose
48. What scoring system can be used in evaluating patients who may have necrotizing fasciitis?
    - ➤ LRINEC (Laboratory Risk Indicator for Necrotizing Fasciitis)
49. What six laboratory markers are needed to calculate the LRINEC score?
    - ➤ CRP ≥150 (4 points)
    - ➤ WBC
        - <15 (0 points)
        - 15-25 (1 point)
        - >25 (2 points)
    - ➤ Hemoglobin
        - >13.5 (0 points)
        - 11-13.5 (1 point)
        - <11 (2 points)

- Sodium <135 (2 points)
- Creatinine >141 (2 points)
- Glucose >180 (1 point)

50. A LRINEC score of what indicates a 92% positive predictive value of having necrotizing fasciitis?
    - ≥ 6
51. What is the most common single isolated organism in necrotizing fasciitis?
    - Group A streptococcus
        - Polymicrobial infections are the most common overall
52. What bacteria is commonly responsible for indolent infections in the shoulder?
    - Propionibacterium acnes
53. How long should cultures be held if there is concern for P. acnes infection?
    - 14-28 days
54. What is pyogenic flexor tenosynovitis?
    - Infection of the synovial sheath surrounding the flexor tendons in the hand
55. What are the Kanavel signs for pyogenic flexor tenosynovitis?
    - Fusiform swelling of the finger
    - Flexed posturing of the finger
    - Tenderness over the length of the flexor sheath
    - Pain with passive extension of the finger
56. What is a horseshoe abscess?
    - Infection of the deep hand connecting the thumb and small finger through Parona's space
57. What is a Paronychia?

The Basics

> Infection of the nail fold

58. Paronychia are most common on which digit?
    > Thumb
59. What is a felon?
    > Infection of the fingertip pulp
60. What is the most common causative organism for paronychias and felons?
    > S. aureus
61. What is a collar button abscess?
    > An abscess of the web space between fingers
62. What is a fight bite injury?
    > Soft tissue injury overlying the dorsal metacarpophalangeal joint, usually from penetration of a tooth
63. What organism is highly associated with fight bite injuries?
    > Eikenella corrodens
64. Are simple dog or cat bites more concerning for development of deep infections?
    > Cat bites
65. What organism is highly associated with cat bite injuries?
    > Pasteurella multocida
66. Septic arthritis most commonly occurs in which joints?
    > Knee > Hip > Shoulder > Elbow > Ankle
67. What is the most common causative organism in septic arthritis?
    > S. aureus

The Basics

68. What bacteria should be considered in a teenage patient with septic arthritis?
    ➢ Neisseria gonorrhea
69. How many WBCs from the aspirate of a native knee suggests septic arthritis?
    ➢ >50,000
70. How many WBCs from a TKA aspirate suggests infection?
    ➢ >1,100
71. How many WBCs from a THA aspirate suggests infection?
    ➢ >3,000
72. What organism is associated with osteomyelitis of the foot following a puncture wound through a shoe?
    ➢ Pseudomonas
73. What bacteria is associated with infections in IV drug abusers?
    ➢ Pseudomonas
74. What bacteria is associated with infections in sickle cell patients?
    ➢ Salmonella

The Basics
Compartment Syndrome

75. What are the six Ps of compartment syndrome?
    - Pain out of proportion
    - Pain with passive stretch
    - Paresthesia
    - Paralysis
    - Pulselessness
    - Poikilothermia
76. What is the most sensitive finding for compartment syndrome on physical exam?
    - Pain with passive stretch
77. What are the compartments of the upper arm?
    - Anterior and Posterior
78. What are the compartments of the forearm?
    - Anterior, Posterior, and Mobile wad
79. What structures are in each compartment of the forearm?
    - Anterior: Pronator teres, Pronator quadratus (PQ), Palmaris longus, FCR, FCU, FDS, FDP, FPL, Radial artery, Ulnar artery, AIN
    - Posterior: Anconeus, EDC, EDM, ECU, Supinator, APL, EPL, EPB, EIP, PIN
    - Mobile Wad: Brachioradialis (BR), ECRL, ECRB, Superficial radial nerve
80. What are the compartments of the hand?
    - Thenar, Hypothenar, Adductor, Dorsal interosseous x4, Volar interosseous x3
81. What are the compartments of thigh?

The Basics

> Anterior, Posterior, and Medial

82. What structures are in each compartment of the thigh?

> Anterior: Quadriceps (Rectus femoris, Vastus lateralis, Vastus medialis, and Vastus intermedius), Articularis genus, Sartorius, Femoral artery and vein, Femoral nerve
> Posterior: Hamstrings (Biceps femoris, Semitendinosus, and Semimembranosus), Sciatic nerve
> Medial: Adductor magnus, Adductor longus, Adductor brevis, Gracilis, Profunda femoris artery and vein, Obturator nerve

83. What are the compartments of the lower leg?

> Anterior, Lateral, Deep posterior, Superficial posterior

84. What structures are in each compartment of the lower leg?

> Anterior: Tibialis anterior, EHL, EDL, Peroneus tertius, Deep peroneal nerve, Anterior tibial artery and vein
> Lateral: Peroneus longus, Peroneus brevis, Superficial peroneal nerve
> Deep posterior: Tibialis posterior, FHL, FDL, Popliteus, Peroneal artery and vein, Tibial nerve, Posterior tibial artery and vein
> Superficial posterior: Gastrocnemius, Soleus, Plantaris

85. What are the compartments of the foot?

- Medial, Lateral, Central superficial, Central deep, Adductor, Interosseous x4

86. Which fracture in adults is the most common cause of acute compartment syndrome?
    - Closed tibial shaft fractures

87. Which fracture in pediatric patients is the most common cause of acute compartment syndrome?
    - Supracondylar humerus fractures

88. What intra-compartmental pressure is suggestive of compartment syndrome?
    - Absolute value ≥30 mmHg
    - Delta P ≤30 mmHg
      - Delta P = Diastolic blood pressure (pre-anesthesia) - Compartment pressure

89. In the setting of a fracture, where should the compartment pressure be measured?
    - Within 5cm of the fracture site

90. What is the treatment for acute compartment syndrome?
    - Emergent fasciotomies

91. Where are the incisions located for a two-incision lower leg fasciotomy?
    - Anterolateral: Half way between the tibial crest and the fibula
    - Medial: Just posterior to the posteromedial border of the tibia

92. Which compartment in the lower leg most commonly develops compartment syndrome?
    - Anterior

The Basics

93. Which compartment is most commonly inadequately released in the lower leg?
    ➢ Deep posterior
94. What condition may occur following missed compartment syndrome of the forearm?
    ➢ Volkmann ischemic contracture

The Basics

General Knowledge

AO/OTA Classification

95. Describe the AO/OTA classification?
    - Type A: Extraarticular fracture
    - Type B: Partial articular fracture
    - Type C: Articular fracture

96. How are the bones numbered in the AO/OTA classification?
    - Humerus: 1
    - Radius/Ulnar: 2
    - Femur/Patella: 3
    - Tibia/Fibula: 4
    - Spine: 5
    - Pelvis/Acetabulum: 6
    - Hand: 7
    - Foot: 8

97. How is fracture location subclassified?
    - Proximal 1/3: 1
    - Shaft: 2
    - Distal 1/3: 3

98. How would you classify a simple, extraarticular midshaft femur fracture using the AO/OTA classification?
    - 32A
        - 3-Femur; 2-Midshaft; A-Extraarticular

Non-Unions

99. What are the different types of nonunions?
    > Atrophic, oligotrophic, hypertrophic, infectious
100. What causes an atrophic nonunion?
    > Too stiff of a construct (no motion)
    > Metabolic disorders
101. What causes a hypertrophic nonunion?
    > Too much motion at the fracture site
102. What labs should be ordered in the workup of a non-union?
    > Infectious: CBC with differential, ESR, CRP
    > Endocrine: Vitamin D, calcium, TSH, PTH

Closed Fractures

103. What is the classification for soft tissue injuries associated with closed fractures?
    > Oestern and Tscherne Classification
        - Grade I: Negligible soft tissue injury
        - Grade II: Superficial contusion or abrasion with a simple fracture
        - Grade III: Deeper contusion or abrasion with risk of compartment syndrome
        - Grade IV: Significant contusion, muscle destruction, subcutaneous degloving, compartment syndrome, nerve or vascular injury

The Basics

Open Fractures

104. How are open fractures classified?
- Gustilo and Anderson
  - Type I: <1cm open wound, low energy fracture
  - Type II: 1-10cm wound
  - Type III: >10cm wound and/or high energy fracture (ie. segmental, comminuted)
    - IIIA: Adequate soft tissue for coverage (includes split thickness skin grafts)
    - IIIB: Requires free or rotational flap for coverage
    - IIIC: Vascular injury requiring repair

105. When is the Gustilo and Anderson classification determined?
- Intraoperatively

106. What is the most important factor in preventing infection in open fractures?
- Time to IV antibiotics

107. What should be given immediately for every open fracture?
- IV antibiotics
- Tetanus – if not up to date

108. What antibiotic is recommended for a Type I open fracture?
- 1st generation cephalosporin (ie. Ancef)

109. What antibiotic may be added for a Type III open fracture?
- Aminoglycoside (ie. Gentamicin)

110. What antibiotic should be added for farm injuries?
> ➤ Penicillin, to cover for Clostridium

111. What antibiotic should be added for water injuries?
> ➤ Fluoroquinolones

112. Anecdotally, how much irrigation is used for each type of open fracture?
> ➤ Type I – 3L
> ➤ Type II – 6L
> ➤ Type III – 9L

113. What is the most important injury predictor for amputation of the lower extremity?
> ➤ Extent of soft tissue injury

114. How should open fractures be treated in the trauma bay?
> ➤ Irrigate the wound and remove any gross debris
> ➤ Reduce the fracture
> ➤ Cover the wound with saline soaked gauze
> ➤ Immobilize the fracture

Osteoporosis

115. What are the definitions of osteopenia and osteoporosis?
> ➤ Osteopenia: T-score between -1 and -2.5
> ➤ Osteoporosis: T-score < -2.5

116. What is the difference between a T-score and a Z-score?
> ➤ T-score relates to a young matched control
> ➤ Z-score compares same aged individuals

117. Is osteoporosis a quantity or quality problem?

The Basics

> ➢ Quantity problem, mineralization of bone is normal

118. How much bone loss is needed to identify osteoporosis on a plain x-ray?
   ➢ 30%

119. What are the three most common insufficiency fractures?
   ➢ Vertebral body > Hip > Wrist

120. What is the one-year, all-cause mortality rate following an insufficiency hip fracture?
   ➢ 33%

121. What is the mechanism of bisphosphonates?
   ➢ Prevents osteoclast formation at the ruffled border and promotes osteoclast apoptosis

122. What is a complication unique to IV bisphosphonates?
   ➢ Jaw osteonecrosis

123. What fractures are suggestive of long-term bisphosphonate use?
   ➢ Atypical subtrochanteric femur fractures

124. What are the characteristics of an atypical femur fracture?
   ➢ Transverse, thick lateral cortex, medial spike

Cartilage

125. What classification is used for chondromalacia?
   ➢ Outerbridge Classification
      - Grade 0: Normal cartilage
      - Grade I: Softening
      - Grade II: Fissuring

- Grade III: Fissuring to subchondral bone
- Grade IV Exposed subchondral bone

126. What type of cartilage covers articular surfaces?
    - Hyaline cartilage (Type II collagen)

127. How does water content of cartilage differ between aging and osteoarthritis?
    - Water content increase with osteoarthritis and decreases with aging

128. What type of collagen is bone?
    - Type I
        - Remember: b**ONE**

Bone Formation

129. What are the main types of ossification?
    - Enchondral – bone is replaced by cartilage
    - Intramembranous – mesenchymal cells become osteoblast
    - Appositional – osteoblast form new bone on existing bone

130. Physeal growth and callus formation represent what type of ossification?
    - Enchondral

131. How does motion effect callus formation?
    - Increase motion leads to increased callus

132. What are the two types of bone healing?
    - Primary (direct) – no callus formation, cutting cones
    - Secondary (indirect) – callus formation

The Basics

133. What type of bone healing is seen with an intramedullary nail? External fixator? Cast? Bridge plating? Lag screw? Compression plating?
> Primary: Lag screw, compression plating
> Secondary: Intramedullary nail, external fixator, bridge plating, cast

Principles & Properties

134. What is Young's modulus of elasticity?
> Resistance of a material to elastic deformation

135. What material has a modulus most similar to bone?
> Titanium

136. What is Wolff's law?
> Remodeling of bone occurs in response to stress

137. What is the Hueter-Volkmann law?
> Compression inhibits growth of bone and tension stimulates bone growth

138. What is the Bernoulli's effect?
> A decrease in pressure causes an increase in fluid speed (Arthroscopy)

139. What are the two ways in which lag screws are placed?
> Lag by technique – the near cortex is over drilled relative to the far cortex
> Lag by design – the proximal aspect of the screw does not have threads (ie. partially threaded)

140. What is a neutralization plate?
> A plate that prevents torsional strain following lag screw fixation

The Basics

141. What is a bridge plate?
   - A plate that spans the fracture site comminution
142. What is a buttress plate?
   - A plate used to prevent collapse under compressive forces
     - Remember: **B**uttress for Type **B** fractures
143. What is an anti-glide plate?
   - A plate used to prevent superior migration under compressive force
     - Upside-down buttress plate
144. What is the pitch of a screw?
   - The distance between screw threads
145. What is the difference between locking and non-locking screws?
   - Locking screws have threaded heads that "lock" into the plate
146. What is countersinking?
   - Creation of a recesses to allow the screw to sit flush with the surface of the bone
147. What are the benefits of countersinking a screw?
   - Decreased prominence
   - Increased surface area for friction between the screw and the bone
148. Bone is strongest and weakest in which planes of motion?
   - Strongest: Compression
   - Weakest: Shear

The Basics

149. What is the classification for nerve injuries?
    - Seddon Classification
        - Neuropraxia: Focal nerve compression
        - Axonotmesis: Axon and myelin disruption with an intact endoneurium
        - Neurotmesis: Complete nerve transection
150. Nerve regeneration occurs at what rate?
    - 1mm/day

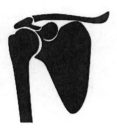

SHOULDER GIRDLE

Shoulder Girdle

General Anatomy

151. What structures make up the superior shoulder suspensory complex?
> Glenoid, Coracoid process, Coracoclavicular ligaments, Distal clavicle, Acromioclavicular joint, Acromial process

152. What are the rotator cuff muscles and their innervations?
> Supraspinatus – Suprascapular nerve
> Infraspinatus – Suprascapular nerve
> Teres minor – Axillary nerve
> Subscapularis – Upper and Lower subscapular nerves

153. What are the borders of the rotator interval?
> Superior – Supraspinatus
> Inferior – Subscapularis
> Medial – Coracoid
> Lateral – Transverse humeral ligament

154. What structures are located within the rotator interval?
> Superior glenohumeral ligament, Long head of the biceps tendon, Coracohumeral ligament, Capsule

155. What is the main bloody supply to the humeral head?
> Posterior humeral circumflex artery

156. Which tendons attach to the greater tuberosity?
> Supraspinatus, Infraspinatus, and Teres minor

157. What tendon attaches to the lesser tuberosity?

Shoulder Girdle

> Subscapularis

158. What structure separates the greater and lesser tuberosities?
    > Bicipital groove
159. What structure attaches just lateral to the bicipital groove?
    > Pectoralis major
160. What structures attach just medial to the bicipital groove?
    > Latissimus dorsi and Teres major
161. Where does the long head of the biceps originate?
    > Supraglenoid tubercle and Superior labrum
162. What structure lies within the deltopectoral interval?
    > Cephalic vein
163. In the deltopectoral approach, what vessels are encountered at the distal margin of the subscapularis tendon?
    > Anterior humeral circumflex artery and its two venous communicantes – "3 Sisters"
164. What structures make up the conjoined tendon?
    > Shorts head of the biceps and Coracobrachialis
165. Which tendons attach to the coracoid?
    > Short head of the biceps, Coracobrachialis, and Pectoralis minor
166. Which ligaments attach to the coracoid?
    > Conoid, Trapezoid, Coracohumeral ligament, and Coracoacromial ligament
167. Which ligaments provide superior and inferior stability to the clavicle?

Shoulder Girdle

➢ Coracoclavicular (CC) – Conoid and Trapezoid

168. Which ligaments provide anterior and posterior stability to the clavicle?

➢ Acromioclavicular (AC)

169. Where do the CC ligaments attach on the clavicle?

➢ Trapezoid: 3cm medial to the AC joint
➢ Conoid: 4.5cm medial to the AC joint

170. Which CC ligament is more posterior?

➢ Conoid

171. Which nerve is at risk with dissection medial to the conjoined tendon?

➢ Musculocutaneous nerve

172. What artery runs along the lateral border of the bicipital groove?

➢ Arcuate artery

173. What percentage of shoulder motion is attributable to the glenohumeral joint and scapulothoracic articulations?

➢ Glenohumeral: 2/3 – 120°
➢ Scapulothoracic: 1/3 – 60°

174. Weakness of which muscle causes medial scapular winging?

➢ Serratus anterior

175. Injury to which nerve causes medial scapular winging?

➢ Long thoracic nerve

176. Weakness of which muscle causes lateral scapular winging?

➢ Trapezius

Shoulder Girdle

177. Injury to which nerve causes lateral scapular winging?
   - Cranial nerve XI

178. The axillary nerve is approximately how far distal to the lateral edge of the acromion?
   - 5cm

179. What are the two predominate heads of the pectoralis major?
   - Clavicular and Sternocostal
     - Sternocostal is most commonly injured

180. Which muscles attach to the scapula?
   - 17 muscles – Supraspinatus, Infraspinatus, Subscapularis, Teres minor, Teres major, Rhomboid major, Rhomboid minor, Levator scapulae, Deltoid, Latissimus dorsi, Serratus anterior, Serratus posterior, Pectoralis minor, Coracobrachialis, Biceps, Triceps, Omohyoid

181. What are the borders of the quadrilateral space?
   - Superior – Teres minor
   - Inferior – Teres major
   - Lateral – Humerus
   - Medial – Long head of the triceps

182. What structures are within the quadrilateral space?
   - Axillary nerve and the Posterior humeral circumflex artery

183. A cyst in the suprascapular notch affects which nerve and muscle(s)?
   - Suprascapular nerve
   - Supraspinatus and Infraspinatus

Shoulder Girdle

184. A cyst in the spinoglenoid notch affects which nerve and muscle(s)?
    - ➤ Suprascapular nerve
    - ➤ Infraspinatus only

185. What is the relationship of the neurovascular structures to the transverse scapular ligament in the suprascapular notch?
    - ➤ Suprascapular artery is above the ligament
    - ➤ Suprascapular nerve is below the ligament
        - Remember: "**A**rtery is **A**bove" or "**A**rmy over **N**avy"

186. What are the primary ligamentous restraints of the shoulder in 0°, 45°, and 90° of abduction?
    - ➤ 0°: Superior glenohumeral ligament (SGHL)
    - ➤ 45°: Middle glenohumeral ligament (MGHL)
    - ➤ 90°: Inferior glenohumeral ligament (IGHL)

187. What is the AP dimension of the supraspinatus footprint?
    - ➤ 12mm

188. Which neurovascular structures are at risk when debriding too medial in the subacromial space during shoulder arthroscopy?
    - ➤ Suprascapular nerve and artery

189. Which vascular structure may be injured with debridement of the coracoacromial ligament?
    - ➤ Acromial branch of the Thoracoacromial artery

190. How far is the top of the greater tuberosity from the pectoralis major tendon?
    - ➤ 5.6cm

Shoulder Girdle

191. Which bone is the first to ossify and the last to fuse?
    - Clavicle

Shoulder Girdle

Trauma

Clavicle

192. What is the classification for lateral third clavicle fractures?
> ➤ Allman/Neer Classification
>   - Type I: Fracture lateral to the CC ligaments
>   - Type II:
>   - A: Fracture medial to the CC ligaments
>   - B1: Fracture between the CC ligaments, conoid torn
>   - B2: Fracture lateral to the CC ligaments, conoid and trapezoid torn
>   - Type III: Fracture extends into the AC joint
>   - Type IV: Physeal fracture
>   - Type V: Comminuted fracture

193. Which part of the clavicle is most commonly fractured?
> ➤ Middle third (80%)

194. What are the deforming forces on each fragment in a middle third clavicle fracture?
> ➤ Sternocleidomastoid muscle pulls the medial fragment posterior and superior
> ➤ Pectoralis major pulls the lateral fragment inferior and medial

195. What are the operative indications for clavicle fractures?

Shoulder Girdle

> Open fractures, skin tenting, neurovascular injuries, Z-deformity, floating shoulder, >2cm shortening, and 100% displacement

196. What are the two plate positions for ORIF of the clavicle?
    > Superior or anterior plating

197. Which plate position is biomechanically stronger?
    > Superior

198. What is the most common patient complaint following superior plating?
    > Hardware prominence

199. What muscle must you split when approaching the clavicle?
    > Platysma
        - Innervated by Cranial nerve VII (Facial)

200. What superficial nerves should you attempt to preserve during the approach to the clavicle?
    > Supraclavicular nerves

201. What defines a floating shoulder?
    > Ipsilateral clavicle and scapula fractures

202. What radiograph should be obtained in PACU following ORIF of the clavicle?
    > Chest x-ray to evaluate for pneumothorax

Acromioclavicular (AC) Joint

203. What is the classification for AC joint injuries?
    > Rockwood Classification
        - Type I: AC sprain
        - Type II: AC ligament tear without CC ligament injury, no displacement

Shoulder Girdle

- Type III: AC and CC ligaments torn, <100% superior displacement of the clavicle
- Type IV: AC and CC ligaments torn, posterior displacement of the clavicle
- Type V: AC and CC ligaments torn, >100% superior displacement of the clavicle
- Type VI: AC and CC ligaments torn, inferior displacement of the clavicle

Scapula

204. What is the classification for scapula fractures?
   - Ideberg
     - Type I: Anterior avulsion
     - Type II: Oblique, exits the glenoid inferiorly
     - Type III: Oblique, exits the glenoid superiorly
     - Type IV: Transverse, exits through the scapular body
     - Type V: Types II + IV

205. What other injuries are highly associated with scapular fractures?
   - Chest wall injuries, lung contusions

Proximal Humerus

206. What is the most widely used classification for proximal humerus fractures?
   - Neer Classification, described by the number of parts

207. What anatomic structures are considered parts?
   - Humeral head, Greater tuberosity, Lesser tuberosity, Humeral shaft

Shoulder Girdle

208. What defines a "part"?
     - ≥45° of angulation and/or ≥1cm of displacement

209. What are the operative indications for proximal humerus fractures?
     - >5mm of greater tuberosity displacement, head splitting fracture, >2-part fracture in young patients

210. Which nerve is most commonly injured following proximal humerus fractures?
     - Axillary

211. What is the classification for AVN of the proximal humerus?
     - Cruess Classification
       - Stage I: Normal on x-ray, changes on MRI
       - Stage II: Sclerosis, osteopenia
       - Stage III: Crescent sign
       - Stage IV: Flattening and collapse
       - Stage V: Degenerative changes of the glenoid

212. What fracture characteristic is a good prognostic indicator for maintaining proximal humerus vascularity?
     - ≥8mm of intact medial calcar on the articular segment

213. What is the most common complication of ORIF for proximal humerus fractures?
     - Screw penetration into the joint

214. What is the most common resultant deformity following failed ORIF of proximal humerus fractures?
     - Varus

Shoulder Girdle

215. What are the two most common surgical approaches to the proximal humerus?
- ➢ Deltopectoral
- ➢ Lateral deltoid split

216. Which structure is at risk during the lateral deltoid split approach?
- ➢ Axillary nerve

Shoulder Dislocations

217. Shoulder dislocations most commonly occur in which direction?
- ➢ Anterior

218. Seizures and electrocution injuries are associated with dislocations in which direction?
- ➢ Posterior

219. Why do these mechanisms increase the risk of posterior dislocation?
- ➢ Internal rotators are more powerful than the external rotators

220. Persistent abduction of the arm is suggestive of a shoulder dislocation in which direction?
- ➢ Inferior
  - ▪ Luxatio Erecta

221. What patient factor is most associated with the risk of recurrent shoulder dislocations?
- ➢ Patient age
  - ▪ <20 years old – 90% chance of redislocation

222. What associated injury should be expected in elderly patients with a shoulder dislocation?
- ➢ Rotator cuff tear

Shoulder Girdle

223. What associated injury should be expected in younger patients with a shoulder dislocation?
    ➤ Instability (ie. Bankart lesions)

224. What humeral sided radiographic finding may be seen following a shoulder dislocation?
    ➤ Hill Sachs lesion

225. Where on the humeral head are Hill Sachs lesions found?
    ➤ Posterosuperior

226. What is the most common nerve injury following a shoulder dislocation?
    ➤ Axillary neuropraxia

Shoulder Girdle

Sports

Rotator Cuff

227. How are rotator cuff tear sizes classified?
    - ➤ DeOrio and Colfield Classification
        - Small: <1cm
        - Medium: 1-3cm
        - Large: 3-5cm
        - Massive: >5cm or ≥2 tendons involved
228. How is rotator cuff atrophy classified?
    - ➤ Goutallier Classification
        - Grade 0: Normal
        - Grade I: Fatty streaking
        - Grade II: More muscle than fat
        - Grade III: Equal amounts of fat and muscle
        - Grade IV: More fat than muscle
229. What is the classification for the shape of the acromion?
    - ➤ Bigliani Classification
        - Type I: Flat
        - Type II: Curved
        - Type III: Hooked
230. The standard anterior portal during shoulder arthroscopy enters the joint through which anatomic area?
    - ➤ Rotator interval
231. Medial subluxation of the long head of the biceps tendon is associated with what pathology?
    - ➤ Subscapularis tendon tear

Shoulder Girdle

232. What physical exam tests are used to evaluate each muscle of the rotator cuff?
- Supraspinatus: Empty can test, drop arm test
- Infraspinatus: External rotation test
- Teres Minor: Hornblowers test
- Subscapularis: Belly press, lift off test

233. What is the rate limiting step in recovery following arthroscopic rotator cuff repair?
- Healing of the repaired tendon to the humerus

234. What is rotator cuff arthropathy?
- Degenerative joint disease secondary to rotator cuff insufficiency

235. What radiographic finding is suggestive of rotator cuff arthropathy?
- Superior head migration

236. What procedure can be performed for an irreparable rotator cuff tear to help prevent superior migration of the humeral head?
- Superior Capsular Reconstruction (SCR)

237. How does failure of a rotator cuff repair most commonly occur?
- Tissue pulls out of the suture

238. What is a PASTA lesion?
- **P**artial **A**rticular **S**upraspinatus **T**endon **A**vulsion

239. What is a Mumford procedure?
- Distal clavicle excision

240. How much distal clavicle may be removed without introducing instability?
- 1cm

Shoulder Girdle

241. What structure should be preserved when performing a Mumford?
> Posterior and superior AC ligaments

Shoulder Instability & Labrum

242. What is a SLAP lesion?
> **S**uperior **L**abral tear – **A**nterior to **P**osterior

243. How are SLAP lesions classified?
> Snyder Classification
> - Type I: Fraying of the superior labrum with an intact bicep anchor
> - Type II: Detachment of the superior labrum and biceps anchor
> - Type III: Bucket-handle tear of the superior labrum with an intact bicep anchor
> - Type IV: Bucket-handle tear of the superior labrum with extension into bicep tendon, anchor detached

244. Which type of SLAP tear is most common?
> Type II

245. Though controversial, patients less than what age are generally candidates for SLAP repairs?
> <40 years old
> - Generally speaking, patients >40 years old typically undergo bicep tenodesis or tenotomy rather than SLAP repair

246. A paralabral cyst on MRI is indicative of what pathology?
> Labral tear

Shoulder Girdle

247. What nerve is at risk with arthroscopic SLAP repair?
    - Suprascapular nerve
248. What is the eponym for an incomplete and usually concealed avulsion of the posterior inferior labrum?
    - Kim lesion
249. Injuries to what part of the labrum are commonly seen in football lineman?
    - Posterior
250. What is the eponym for an absent anterosuperior labrum with a cordlike MGHL?
    - Buford Complex
251. What happens if an unrecognized Buford Complex is "repaired"?
    - Shoulder tightness – loss of external rotation and elevation
252. Define "TUBS"
    - **T**raumatic, **U**nilateral dislocation, **B**ankart, **S**urgery required
253. Define "AMBRI"
    - **A**traumatic, **M**ultidirectional, **B**ilateral, **R**esponds to **R**ehab, **I**nferior capsular shift
254. What is a "drive through sign"?
    - Ability to pass arthroscope easily between the humeral head and the glenoid inferiorly suggesting shoulder laxity
255. What is a Bankart lesion?
    - Anterior inferior labral tear
256. Where is the fracture located in a "bony Bankart"?
    - Anterior inferior glenoid

Shoulder Girdle

257. What is a HAGL lesion?
- ➢ **H**umeral **A**vulsion of the **G**lenohumeral **L**igament
  - Anterior inferior glenohumeral ligament

258. What is a GLAD lesion?
- ➢ **G**lenoid **L**abral **A**rticular **D**efect

259. What is an ALPSA lesions?
- ➢ **A**nterior **L**abral **P**eriosteal **S**leeve **A**vulsion

260. What is the apprehension sign on physical exam?
- ➢ Patient becomes apprehensive with shoulder abduction and external rotation
  - Sensation relieved with posterior force placed on the anterior shoulder (Relocation test)

261. What is a Latarjet procedure?
- ➢ Coracoid transfer to the anterior glenoid

262. What percentage of glenoid bone loss is an indication to perform a Latarjet?
- ➢ 20%

263. What is a Remplissage?
- ➢ Suturing the posterior capsule and infraspinatus tendon into a Hill Sachs lesion

Proximal Biceps

264. What two physical exam maneuvers are used to test the proximal biceps?
- ➢ Speed: Shoulder forward flexed to 90°, elbow extended, forearm supinated
  - Pain with resisted elevation
- ➢ Yergason: Arm by the patient's side, elbow flexed to 90°

- Pain with resisted forearm supination and external rotation

265. What are the two surgical options for a diseased proximal biceps tendon?
    - Biceps tenotomy or tenodesis

266. What is the difference in strength following biceps tenotomy when compared to tenodesis?
    - None, weakness is not associated with biceps tenotomy

267. What complaints do patients typically have following biceps tenotomy without tenodesis?
    - Cramping
    - Cosmetic Popeye deformity

Adhesive Capsulitis & GIRD

268. What is GIRD?
    - **G**leno**h**umeral **I**nternal **R**otation **D**eficit caused by posteroinferior capsular tightening

269. What sporting activity most commonly leads to GIRD?
    - Pitching in baseball

270. What stretch is the mainstay of treatment?
    - Sleeper stretch

271. What do you see on physical exam with adhesive capsulitis (frozen shoulder)?
    - Significant loss of both active and passive shoulder range of motion

272. Which structures are primarily affected in adhesive capsulitis?
    - Coracohumeral ligament

Shoulder Girdle

> Rotator interval

273. What motion is most restricted in adhesive capsulitis?

> External rotation

274. What MR arthrogram finding indicates contracture of the joint capsule?

> Loss of the axillary recess

275. Is adhesive capsulitis more common in men or women?

> Women

276. What two medical conditions have a strong association with adhesive capsulitis?

> Diabetes and hypothyroidism

Adult Reconstruction

Shoulder Hemiarthroplasty

277. What is another prosthetic alternative to reverse total shoulder arthroplasty (RSA) in a young active patient with rotator cuff arthropathy and preserved shoulder motion?
    - Hemiarthroplasty
        - Cuff Tear Arthropathy (CTA) components

278. What is the most important factor affecting function following hemiarthroplasty?
    - Rotator cuff function

279. What is the most common indication for revision following a shoulder hemiarthroplasty in a young patient?
    - Glenoid erosion

280. When treating a proximal humerus fracture with shoulder hemiarthroplasty, what is the most common complication?
    - Greater and lesser tuberosity malunion, non-union, or resorption

Total Shoulder Arthroplasty (TSA)

281. How is wear of the glenoid classified?
    - Walch Classification
        - Type A: Central erosion
            - A1: Minor
            - A2: Deep

Shoulder Girdle

- Type B: Posterior subluxation of the humeral head
  - B1: Posterior glenoid wear
  - B2: Biconcave glenoid wear
  - B3: Progression of biconcave wear to >80%
- Type C: >25° of glenoid retroversion (associated with glenoid dysplasia)

282. What glenoid wear pattern is more common with rheumatoid arthritis?
   ➤ Central wear

283. What glenoid wear pattern is more common with osteoarthritis?
   ➤ Posterior wear

284. What are contraindications for TSA?
   ➤ Rotator cuff arthropathy, irreparable rotator cuff tear, inadequate bone stock, infection

285. What is the most commonly used surgical approach for TSA?
   ➤ Deltopectoral

286. The humeral head is retroverted how many degrees relative to the transepicondylar axis?
   ➤ 20-30°

287. How much glenoid retroversion can be correct with reaming?
   ➤ 15°

288. What is the "Rocking Horse" phenomenon?
   ➤ Loosening of the glenoid component due to edge loading

289. With what pathology is the "Rocking Horse" phenomenon seen?

> Rotator cuff insufficiency

290. Which nerve is at risk with a retractor placed under the conjoint tendon?
    > Musculocutaneous

291. What motion should be restricted in the first 6 weeks following TSA?
    > External rotation to protect the subscapularis tendon repair

Reverse Shoulder Arthroplasty (RSA)

292. What are the indications for a primary RSA?
    > Rotator cuff tear arthropathy, rheumatoid arthritis, failed TSA, 3 and 4-part proximal humerus fractures in elderly patients, B2 glenoid osteoarthritis in the elderly

293. What are the contraindications to RSA?
    > Axillary nerve dysfunction, acromion deficiency

294. Where should the glenosphere be placed in a Grammont style RSA?
    > As inferiorly on the glenoid as possible with inferior tilt

295. What is the most common complication that occurs if the glenosphere is malpositioned superiorly?
    > Scapular notching

296. What is the classification for scapular notching?
    > Sirveaux Classification
    >   - Grade I: Notching to scapular pillar
    >   - Grade II: Notching to the inferior screw of the baseplate

Shoulder Girdle

- Grade III: Notching beyond the inferior screw of the baseplate
- Grade IV: Notching to the central peg of the baseplate

297. What fracture must be ruled out after a fall in a patient with a RSA?

> Acromion fracture

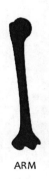

ARM

Arm

General Anatomy

298. How far proximal is the radial nerve from the medial and lateral epicondyles?
    - Medial: 20cm
    - Lateral: 14cm
299. The radial nerve can be found between what two muscles on the anterolateral arm?
    - Brachialis and Brachioradialis
300. What are the two terminal branches of the radial nerve?
    - Superficial radial nerve, Posterior interosseous nerve (PIN)
301. Where does the radial nerve division occur?
    - At the level of the radial head
302. Following a radial nerve injury, what is the last muscle to regain function?
    - Extensor indicis proprius (EIP)
303. What is the innervation of the brachialis muscle?
    - Lateral 1/3: Radial nerve
    - Medial 2/3: Musculocutaneous nerve
304. What is the terminal branch of the musculocutaneous nerve?
    - Lateral antebrachial cutaneous nerve
305. At what level does the ulnar nerve travel from the anterior to posterior compartment?
    - At the arcade of Struthers
        - 8 cm proximal to the medial epicondyle
306. What are the 3 heads of the triceps muscle?
    - Lateral, long, and medial

307. Where does the long head of the triceps originate?
   ➤ Inferior glenoid tubercle

Arm

Trauma

Humerus

308. What are the classifications for single and two column distal humerus fractures?
   - Milch Classification (single column fractures)
     - Type I: Lateral trochlear ridge intact
     - Type II: Fracture through the lateral trochlear ridge
   - Jupiter classification (two column fractures)
     - Descriptive: High-T, Low-T, Y, H, Lambda

309. What is a Holstein-Lewis fracture?
   - Spiral, distal 1/3 humerus fracture with associated radial nerve palsy

310. What are the nonoperative tolerances for humeral shaft fractures?
   - Coronal plane: <30°
   - Sagittal plane: <20°
   - Shortening: <3cm

311. What type of splint is initially used for midshaft humerus fractures?
   - Coaptation splint

312. What type of mold should be placed on a coaptation splint?
   - Valgus mold

313. What brace can be used for nonoperative treatment of a humeral shaft fracture?
   - Functional (Sarmiento) brace

314. How does a functional brace work?
   - Hydrostatic pressure maintains reduction

315. Is a radial nerve palsy a contraindication to functional bracing?
   ➢ No

316. With humeral nailing, which nerve is at risk when placing a distal anterior to posterior screw?
   ➢ Musculocutaneous nerve

317. With humeral nailing, which nerve is at risk when placing a distal lateral to medial screw?
   ➢ Radial nerve

318. What are the treatment options for a comminuted distal humerus fracture in an elderly, low demand patient?
   ➢ Nonoperative, ORIF, Total Elbow Arthroplasty (TEA)

319. What fracture is a relative contraindication to TEA?
   ➢ Olecranon fracture

320. Are there any permanent postoperative restrictions following TEA?
   ➢ Refrain from repetitive lifting >5 pounds

321. What are the O'Driscoll principles for ORIF of distal humerus fractures?
   ➢ As many screws as possible should be placed in the distal fragments
   ➢ Every screw in the distal fragments should pass through a plate
   ➢ Every screw should be as long as possible
   ➢ Every screw should engage as many articular fragments as possible

Arm

- Screws should engage a fragment on the opposite side
- Screws should be interdigitated
- Plates are positioned such that compression is obtained at the supracondylar level for both columns

322. What distal humerus approach allows for direct visualization of the joint surface?

- Posterior approach with an olecranon osteotomy

323. What is the shape of the olecranon osteotomy?

- Distal chevron

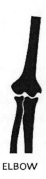

ELBOW

Elbow

General Anatomy

324. What is the functional range of motion of the elbow?
   ➢ 30-130° of flexion
   ➢ 50° of both supination and pronation
325. What is the normal carrying angle of the elbow?
   ➢ 10-15° of valgus
326. The capsule of the elbow is maximally distended at what degree of flexion?
   ➢ 75°
327. What structures create the borders of the "soft spot" on the lateral aspect of the elbow?
   ➢ Olecranon, Lateral epicondyle, and Radial head
328. What muscles originate on the medial epicondyle?
   ➢ PT, FCR, PL, FDS, FCU
329. What muscles originate on the lateral epicondyle?
   ➢ Anconeus, ECRL ECRB, EDC EDM, ECU
330. Where does the medial collateral ligament of the elbow insert?
   ➢ Sublime tubercle
331. Is the MCL tighter in pronation or supination?
   ➢ Pronation
332. What are the bundles of the MCL?
   ➢ Anterior, posterior, and transverse
333. Which bundle of the MCL is the primary restraint to valgus motion?
   ➢ Anterior
334. What 4 structures make up the lateral collateral ligament complex?

Elbow

- Lateral (radial) collateral ligament (LCL)
- Accessory LCL
- Lateral ulnar collateral ligament (LUCL)
- Annular ligament

335. Where does the LUCL insert?
- Crista supinatorus (Supinator Crest)

336. Is the LUCL tighter in pronation or supination?
- Supination

337. What is the primary stabilizer to varus and external rotation stress of the elbow?
- LUCL

338. What structure is at risk with dissection distal to the annular ligament?
- Posterior interosseous nerve (PIN)

339. What is the interval for the Kaplan approach?
- EDC (PIN) and ECRB (Radial nerve)

340. What is the interval for the Kocher approach?
- ECU (PIN) and Anconeus (Radial nerve)

341. What nerve is at greatest risk with the Kaplan and Kocher approaches?
- PIN

342. How should the forearm be positioned to minimize risk to the PIN during the Kaplan or Kocher approach?
- Pronated

343. What are the six entrapment sites of the ulnar nerve about the elbow?
- Arcade of Struthers

Elbow

- Remember: **A**rcade and **U**lnar both start with vowels. Do not confuse with the Ligament of Struthers
- Medial head of the triceps
- Medial intermuscular septum
- Osbourne's ligament
- Anconeus epitrochlearis
- Two heads of the FCU

344. What is the most common site for ulnar nerve entrapment about the elbow?

- Between the two heads of the FCU

345. What physical exam finding is present with ulnar nerve compression about the elbow, but not present with compression distally in Guyon's canal?

- Sensory deficits over the dorsal lateral hand

346. What are the five entrapment sites of the radial nerve about the elbow?

- Fibrous bands around the radial head
- Leash of Henry
- Arcade of Frohse
- Distal aspect of the supinator muscle
- ECRB

347. What is the most common site for radial nerve entrapment about the elbow?

- Arcade of Frohse

348. What is the Arcade of Frohse?

- Proximal edge of the supinator muscle

349. What are the five entrapment sites of the median nerve about the elbow?

- Supracondylar process

Elbow

> Ligament of Struthers
> Bicipital aponeurosis
> Two heads of the pronator teres
> FDS

350. What is the most common site for median nerve entrapment about the elbow?
> Between the two heads of pronator teres

351. What cutaneous nerve is commonly encountered during a cubital tunnel release?
> Medial antebrachial cutaneous nerve

352. What are the first two branches of the ulnar nerve after it passes into the posterior compartment?
> First branch: Articular branch
> Second branch: Nerve to FCU

353. Which nerve is at risk when placing the proximal anterolateral portal for elbow arthroscopy?
> Radial nerve

354. Which nerve is at risk when placing the distal anterolateral portal for elbow arthroscopy?
> Lateral antebrachial cutaneous

355. Which nerve is at risk when placing the proximal anteromedial portal for elbow arthroscopy?
> Medial antebrachial cutaneous

356. What is the primary function of the long head of the biceps?
> Supination

357. Where on the radial tuberosity does the biceps tendon insert?
> Ulnar aspect

Elbow

358. Which head of the biceps inserts more proximally on the radial tuberosity?
    ➤ Long head
359. What is the interval for a distal biceps repair?
    ➤ Pronator Teres (Median nerve) and Brachioradialis (Radial nerve)

Trauma

Capitellum & Trochlea

360. What is the classification for capitellum fractures?
    - Bryan and Morrey Classification
        - Type I: Large osseous piece
        - Type II: Shear fracture of articular surface (Kocher-Lorenz)
        - Type III: Comminuted (Broberg-Morrey)
        - Type IV: Coronal shear of capitellum and trochlea

361. What is the most common complication following ORIF of fractures about the elbow?
    - Elbow stiffness

Proximal Ulna

362. What is the classification for coronoid fractures?
    - Regan Morrey Classification
        - Type 1: Coronoid tip fractures
        - Type 2: Fracture involving <50% of coronoid height
        - Type 3: Fracture involving >50% of coronoid height
    - O'Driscoll Classification
        - Descriptive of fracture location and number of fracture fragments
            - Tip
            - Anteromedial facet
            - Basal

Elbow

363. What injury should be considered with a coronoid fracture?
    ➢ Elbow dislocation
364. What is a Monteggia fracture?
    ➢ Proximal ulna fracture with a radial head dislocation
365. What is the classification for Monteggia fractures?
    ➢ Bado classification
        - Type I: Anterior radial head dislocation and apex anterior proximal ulna fracture
        - Type II: Posterior radial head dislocation and apex posterior proximal ulna fracture
        - Type III: Lateral radial head dislocation and apex lateral proximal ulna fracture
        - Type IV: Fractures of the proximal radius and ulna with radial head dislocation
366. Which nerve is most at risk with a Monteggia fracture?
    ➢ PIN
367. What commonly leads to continued radial head dislocation following ulnar fixation in a Monteggia fracture?
    ➢ Malreduction of the ulna

Proximal Radius

368. What is the classification for radial head fractures?
    ➢ Mason Classification
        - Type I: <2mm displacement
        - Type II: >2mm displacement
        - Type III: Comminuted

Elbow

- Type IV: Radial head fracture with an elbow dislocation

369. Interposition of what structure may lead to an irreducible radiocapitellar joint?
    ➢ Annular ligament

370. What quadrant of the radial head is most vulnerable to fracture?
    ➢ Anterolateral

371. What are the surgical treatment options for radial head fractures?
    ➢ ORIF, replacement, and excision

372. Where is the non-articular portion of the radial head located?
    ➢ 90° arc from Listers tubercle to the radial styloid

373. Why is the non-articular portion of the radial head important?
    ➢ Safe zone for hardware placement

Elbow

Sports

Elbow Instability

374. What is the terrible triad of the elbow?
   ➤ Coronoid fracture, radial head fracture, and elbow dislocation
375. What is the circle of Hori?
   ➤ The ligaments of the elbow fail from lateral to medial
   ➤ LCL → Capsule → MCL
376. Where do LCL injuries most commonly occur?
   ➤ Proximally as avulsions off the lateral epicondyle
377. Injury to the LUCL leads to what type of elbow instability?
   ➤ Posterolateral rotatory instability
378. Fracture of what percentage of the coronoid may result in instability?
   ➤ >50%
379. What type of instability is associated with an anteromedial coronoid fracture and LCL injury?
   ➤ Varus posteromedial rotatory instability
380. What stabilizes the proximal radioulnar joint?
   ➤ Annular ligament
381. In which direction does the elbow most commonly dislocate?
   ➤ Posterolateral
382. What is the difference between a simple and a complex elbow dislocation?
   ➤ Simple dislocations occur without fractures

Elbow

Epicondylitis

383. What is the eponym for medial epicondylitis?
    ➢ Golfer's elbow
384. What clinical examination test assesses for medial epicondylitis?
    ➢ Resisted wrist flexion and pronation
385. What is the eponym for lateral epicondylitis?
    ➢ Tennis elbow
386. Which tendon is most commonly involved in lateral epicondylitis?
    ➢ ECRB tendon
387. What histologic finding is seen with lateral epicondylitis?
    ➢ Angiofibroblastic dysplasia
388. What clinical examination test assesses for lateral epicondylitis?
    ➢ Resisted wrist extension

Distal Biceps

389. Partial distal biceps tendon tears occur on what side of the radial tuberosity?
    ➢ Radial side
390. What type of muscular contraction commonly leads to distal biceps rupture?
    ➢ Eccentric contraction
391. What deformity may occur following a distal bicep tendon rupture?
    ➢ Reverse Popeye deformity
392. What is the hook test?

Elbow

> Hooking the lateral edge of the bicep tendon with the elbow flexed to 90° and supinated

393. What structure may give a false positive hook test if performed from medial to lateral?

> Lacertus fibrosis

394. What is the first nerve at risk during the approach to repair a distal biceps tendon rupture?

> Lateral antebrachial cutaneous nerve

395. What complications are more common with single and double incision repairs?

> Single incision: Synostosis
> Double incision: Heterotopic ossification

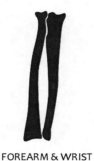

FOREARM & WRIST

Forearm & Wrist

General Anatomy

396. What are the five ligaments of the interosseous membrane?
> - Central band
> - Accessory band
> - Distal oblique bundle
> - Proximal oblique cord
> - Dorsal oblique accessory cord

397. Which ligament of the interosseous membrane is most important for stability?
> - Central band
>   - Second principle stabilizer of the radius

398. What is the relationship of the bicipital tuberosity and the radial styloid on an AP radiograph?
> - 180°

399. What is the relationship of the coronoid and the ulnar styloid on a lateral radiograph?
> - 180°

400. What is the most distal muscle belly on the extensor side of the forearm?
> - Extensor indicis proprius (EIP)

401. What are the components of the triangular fibrocartilage complex (TFCC)?
> - **M**eniscal homologue
> - **A**rticular disc
> - **U**lnolunate and **U**lnotriquetral ligaments
> - **E**CU subsheath
> - **R**adioulnar ligaments – volar and dorsal
>   - Remember: "Dr. **MAUER**"

Forearm & Wrist

402. Which ligaments of the TFCC are the primary stabilizers?
    ➢ Radioulnar ligaments – volar and dorsal

403. In which positions are the radioulnar ligaments of the DRUJ most stable?
    ➢ Dorsal radioulnar ligaments: Supination
    ➢ Volar radioulnar ligaments: Pronation

404. Which nerve innervates the wrist capsule?
    ➢ PIN

405. Which tendon is found directly ulnar to Lister's tubercle?
    ➢ EPL

406. What are the contents of the six extensor compartments of the wrist?
    ➢ 1st – APL, EPB
    ➢ 2nd – ECRL, ECRB
    ➢ 3rd – EPL
    ➢ 4th – EDC, EIP, PIN
    ➢ 5th – EDM
    ➢ 6th – ECU

407. Which 1st extensor compartment tendon has more variable anatomy?
    ➢ APL, which may have multiple slips

408. What condition is associated with the first extensor compartment?
    ➢ Dequervain's tenosynovitis

409. What condition is associated with the second extensor compartment?
    ➢ Intersection syndrome

Forearm & Wrist

410. What is the most common dorsal approach to the distal radius?
> Incise the 3rd extensor compartment with elevation of the radial aspect of the 4th extensor compartment

411. What are the branches of the median nerve at the level of the wrist?
> Median nerve proper, Palmar cutaneous branch, and Recurrent motor branch

412. The palmar cutaneous branch of the median nerve gives sensation to which part of the hand?
> Thenar eminence

413. How much of the weight-bearing force is transmitted through the distal radius and ulna?
> Distal radius: 80%
> Distal ulna: 20%

414. How much of the weight-bearing force is transmitted through the proximal radius and ulna?
> Proximal radius: 60%
> Proximal ulna: 40%

415. Why does the weight-bearing force for the proximal radius and ulna differ from the distal distributions?
> The interosseous membrane distributes more force to the ulna proximally

416. What is the most commonly used surgical approach for the distal radius?
> Volar Henry and its modifications (FCR approach)

417. What is the FCR approach?

Forearm & Wrist

> Incision centered over the FCR tendon. Superficial FCR tendon sheath is incised. FCR retracted. Dorsal FCR sheath is incised. FPL is identified and retracted. Pronator quadratus is detached

418. Which nerve is located under the ulnar border of the FCR sheath?

> Palmar cutaneous branch of the median nerve

419. What is the name of the most common dorsal approach used for middle and proximal 1/3 radius fractures?

> Dorsal Thompson

420. What are the proximal and distal intervals for the Dorsal Thompson approach?

> Proximally: EDC and ECRB
> Distally: ECRB and EPL

421. Which nerve is at risk in the proximal portion of the Dorsal Thompson approach?

> PIN as it traverses the supinator

Forearm & Wrist

Trauma

Forearm

422. What are the operative indications for forearm fractures?
   - ➢ Proximal 1/3 ulna fractures
   - ➢ Displaced distal 2/3 ulna fractures
   - ➢ Displaced radius fractures
   - ➢ Fractures causing a loss of the radial bow
   - ➢ Both bone forearm fractures
   - ➢ Open fractures

423. What are the eponyms for a fracture of the distal radius with an associated DRUJ injury?
   - ➢ Galeazzi fracture, Fracture of necessity, and Piedmont fracture

424. Post-operative forearm function depends on restoration of what during ORIF?
   - ➢ Radial bow

425. The radial head should align with the capitellum on which x-ray views?
   - ➢ All views

426. What complication may occur following ORIF of a both bone forearm fracture through a single incision?
   - ➢ Synostosis

Wrist

427. What are the normal radiographic parameters for radial height, volar tilt, and radial inclination?
   - ➢ Radial height: 11mm

> Volar tilt: 11°
> Radial inclination: 22°

428. Why should a forearm x-ray be obtained in the setting of wrist pain following trauma?
   > To evaluate for an Essex-Lopresti injury pattern

429. What is an Essex-Lopresti fracture?
   > Fracture of the radial head with concomitant disruption of the DRUJ and central band of the interosseous membrane

430. What may occur in an unrecognized Essex-Lopresti fracture?
   > Proximal migration of the radius

431. What neuropathy is associated with a DRUJ injury?
   > Ulnar nerve neuropathy

432. What clinical test is often used to evaluate for DRUJ instability?
   > Shuck test

433. What ligaments are evaluated with the Shuck test?
   > Radioulnar ligaments of the TFCC

434. What structure may lead to an irreducible DRUJ?
   > Interposition of the ECU tendon

435. What is the eponym for a depressed fracture of the lunate fossa?
   > Die-punch fracture

436. What is the eponym for an isolated radial styloid fracture?
   > Chauffeur's fracture

437. What is the eponym for an intra-articular distal radius fracture with dislocation of the radiocarpal joint?

Forearm & Wrist

> ➢ Barton's fracture

438. What is the eponym for an apex volar extra-articular distal radius fracture?

> ➢ Colles' fracture

439. What is the eponym for an apex dorsal extra-articular distal radius fracture?

> ➢ Smith's fracture

440. What acute neuropathy may occur with a distal radius fracture?

> ➢ Acute carpal tunnel – this is a surgical emergency

441. What are the acceptable post-reduction parameters for treating a distal radius fracture nonoperatively?

> ➢ Radial height: <5mm of shortening
> ➢ Volar tilt: Dorsal angulation <5° or within 20° of the contralateral side
> ➢ Radial inclination: <5° difference to contralateral
> ➢ Articular step-off: <2mm

442. What are the modified LaFontaine criteria?

> ➢ Dorsal angulation >20°
> ➢ Dorsal comminution >50%, palmar comminution, intraarticular comminution
> ➢ Initial displacement >1cm
> ➢ Initial radial shortening >5mm
> ➢ Associated ulna fracture
> ➢ Severe osteoporosis or age >60 years

443. How many of the modified LaFontaine criteria suggests an unstable fracture?

> ➢ ≥3

444. Which nerve is at risk with the radial shaft pin of a wrist spanning external fixator?

Forearm & Wrist

445. What distal radius parameter cannot reliably be restored with utilization of a wrist spanning external fixator?
    ➢ Volar tilt

446. Rupture of which tendon is most common following ORIF of the distal radius utilizing a volar approach?
    ➢ FPL

447. How does volar plate placement influence FPL rupture risk?
    ➢ Increased risk of FPL rupture if the plate is placed distal to watershed line

448. Rupture of which tendon is most common following nonoperative management of a distal radius fracture?
    ➢ EPL – due to increased pressure over the watershed area of the tendon around Lister's tubercle or from mechanical attrition due to callus formation

449. What tendon transfer is performed to treat EPL ruptures?
    ➢ EIP to EPL transfer

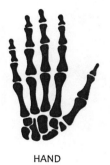

HAND

Hand

General Anatomy

450. What structures make up the borders of the carpal tunnel?
    ➢ Roof: Transverse carpal ligament
    ➢ Floor: Proximal carpal row
    ➢ Ulnar: Hook of hamate and Pisiform
    ➢ Radial: Trapezium and Scaphoid
451. What are the contents of the carpal tunnel?
    ➢ FDS tendons x4
    ➢ FDP tendons x4
    ➢ FPL
    ➢ Median nerve
452. What is the most radial structure within the carpal tunnel?
    ➢ FPL
453. How are the FDS tendons oriented within the carpal tunnel?
    ➢ The tendons to the middle and ring fingers are superficial to the tendons for the index and small fingers
454. Which nerve is occasionally present within the transverse carpal ligament?
    ➢ Recurrent motor branch of the median nerve
455. In what percentage of patients is the recurrent motor branch of the median nerve transligamentous?
    ➢ 20%
456. What is the function of the sagittal band?
    ➢ Keeps the extensor mechanism centered over the digit

Hand

457. What minimizes extensor tendon retraction following rupture?
    ➢ Juncturae tendinum
458. How are the bones of the proximal carpal row orientated from radial to ulnar?
    ➢ **S**caphoid, **L**unate, **T**riquetrum, **P**isiform
        ▪ Remember "**S**o **L**ong **T**o **P**inky"
459. How are the bones of the distal carpal row orientated from ulnar to radial?
    ➢ **H**amate, **C**apitate, **T**rapezoid, **T**rapezium
        ▪ Remember "**H**ere **C**omes **T**he **T**humb"
460. What is the main blood supply to the scaphoid?
    ➢ Dorsal carpal branch of the radial artery
461. What are the borders of the anatomical snuffbox?
    ➢ Ulnar border: EPL
    ➢ Radial border: APL and EPB
    ➢ Proximal border: Radial styloid
462. What structures make up the borders of Guyon's canal?
    ➢ Floor: Transverse carpal ligament
    ➢ Roof: Volar carpal ligament
    ➢ Radial: Hook of the Hamate
    ➢ Ulnar: Pisiform
463. What are the zones of the ulnar nerve as it traverses Guyon's canal?
    ➢ Zone I: Proximal to bifurcation
        ▪ Motor and Sensory
    ➢ Zone II: Deep motor branch
    ➢ Zone III: Superficial sensory branch

Hand

464. What area of the volar palm is susceptible to lunate dislocation?
    - Space of Poirier
465. Where does the FCR tendon insert?
    - Base of the 2nd metacarpal
466. Where does the FCU tendon insert?
    - Pisiform, Hook of hamate, and Base of 5th metacarpal
467. How many compartments are in the hand and what are they?
    - 10 Compartments
        - Hypothenar
        - Thenar
        - Adductor Pollicis
        - Dorsal Interosseous x4
        - Volar Interosseous x3
468. Which nerve is evaluated with the "OK" sign?
    - AIN
469. What muscles are innervated by the AIN?
    - Pronator quadratus
    - FPL
    - FDP to the index and middle fingers
470. Which nerve is evaluated with the "thumbs up" sign?
    - PIN
471. Which nerve is evaluated with adduction and abduction of the fingers?
    - Ulnar nerve
472. Where do the lumbrical muscles originate?
    - FDP tendons

Hand

473. What is the function of the lumbrical muscles?
   ➤ Flexion of the MCP joints and extension of the IP joints

474. What is the relationship of the lumbricals and the interossei to the transverse metacarpal ligament?
   ➤ **L**umbricals are **V**olar
      - Remember: **L**as **V**egas
   ➤ Interossei are dorsal
      - Remember: **ID**

475. Where do the FDS tendons insert?
   ➤ Middle phalanx

476. Which tendon flexes the proximal interphalangeal (PIP) joint?
   ➤ FDS

477. Where do the FDP tendons insert?
   ➤ Distal phalanx

478. Which tendon flexes the distal interphalangeal (DIP) joint?
   ➤ FDP

479. Does FDS or FDP have a common muscle belly in the forearm?
   ➤ FDP

480. What is the name of the anatomic location where the FDP tendon passes through the FDS tendon?
   ➤ Camper's chiasm

481. What is the location of Camper's chiasm?
   ➤ At the level of the proximal phalanx

482. What are the two extensor tendons of the index finger?
   ➤ EDC index and EIP

Hand

483. Which index finger extensor tendon is more ulnar?
    - EIP

484. Which artery primarily supplies the superficial arch of the hand?
    - Ulnar artery

485. Which artery primarily supplies the deep arch of the hand?
    - Radial artery

486. Most commonly, which artery predominately supplies the hand?
    - Ulnar artery

487. Which vascular arch is more distal in the palm?
    - Superficial

488. What is Kaplan's cardinal line?
    - A line extending from the ulnar side of the abducted thumb to the hook of the hamate

489. How far are the superficial and deep palmar arches from Kaplan's cardinal line?
    - Superficial: 15mm distal
    - Deep: 7mm distal

490. How far are the superficial and deep palmar arches from the wrist crease?
    - Superficial: 5cm distal
    - Deep: 4cm distal

491. The digital arteries typically arise from which palmar arch?
    - Superficial

492. What is the relationship between the digital arteries and nerves in the palm?
    - Arteries are volar to the nerves

Hand

493. What is the relationship between the digital arteries and nerves in the digits?
   ➤ Arteries are dorsal to the nerves
494. Which digital artery is predominant?
   ➤ Predominant vessel is closer to midline
     ▪ Index and Middle: Ulnar digital artery
     ▪ Ring and Small: Radial digital artery
495. Which digital cutaneous ligament (Cleland's or Grayson's) is palmar to the digital nerve?
   ➤ Grayson's
     ▪ Remember **CD** (**C**leland's is **D**orsal)
496. Is Cleland's or Grayson's ligament involved in Dupuytren's disease?
   ➤ Grayson's ligament
497. How many pulleys are in the fingers?
   ➤ 8 pulleys
     ▪ 5 annular pulleys
     ▪ 3 cruciate pulleys
498. How are the pulleys of the finger ordered from proximal to distal?
   ➤ A1, A2, C1, A3, C2, A4, C3, A5
499. Which pulleys are located over the MCPJ, PIPJ and DIPJ?
   ➤ MCPJ: A1
   ➤ PIPJ: A3
   ➤ DIPJ: A5
500. Which two pulleys are the most crucial in preventing bowstringing of the fingers?
   ➤ A2 and A4

Hand

501. Where on the finger are the A2 and A4 pulleys located?
    ➢ A2: Proximal aspect of the proximal phalanx
    ➢ A4: Middle aspect of the middle phalanx

502. What is the most important pulley in the thumb?
    ➢ Oblique pulley

503. When evaluating the flexion cascade, the fingertips should all point towards what bony landmark?
    ➢ Scaphoid tubercle

504. Where does the central slip of the finger insert?
    ➢ Dorsal middle phalanx

505. Which structure may prevent the reduction of an interphalangeal joint dislocation?
    ➢ Volar plate

506. Which two ligaments create the ulnar collateral ligament (UCL) of the thumb?
    ➢ Proper and Accessory collateral ligaments

507. Where do the collateral ligaments of the finger insert?
    ➢ Proper: Base of the phalanx
    ➢ Accessory: Volar plate

508. What is a Martin-Gruber anastomosis?
    ➢ Nerve communication between the median and ulnar nerves in the forearm

509. What is a Riches-Cannieu anastomosis?
    ➢ Nerve communication between the recurrent branch of the median nerve and the deep branch of the ulnar nerve in the hand

Hand Conditions

Carpal Tunnel Syndrome

510. What is the most sensitive test for diagnosing carpal tunnel syndrome?
    - Durkan's compression test
511. How do you perform Durkan's compression test?
    - Hold pressure over carpal tunnel for 30 seconds
        - Pain or paresthesia indicate a positive test
512. What are the two ways in which a carpal tunnel release can be performed?
    - Open or endoscopic
513. Which structure may be injured if the transverse carpal ligament is incised too radially?
    - Recurrent motor branch of the median nerve
514. Which muscles demonstrate atrophy with long standing carpal tunnel syndrome?
    - Thenar muscles – Flexor pollicis brevis, Opponens pollicis, and Abductor pollicis brevis
515. What is the most common reason for failed endoscopic carpal tunnel surgery?
    - Incomplete release of the transverse carpal ligament distally
516. Is there any difference in outcomes following open vs endoscopic carpal tunnel release?
    - Patients with endoscopic surgery return to work earlier
    - No difference in long-term patient outcomes

Hand

Scaphoid

517. Following scapholunate ligament disruption, which part of the ligamentous complex must be repaired?
    ➤ Dorsal interosseous ligaments

518. What is unique about the blood supply of the scaphoid?
    ➤ Retrograde blood supply

519. How does the retrograde blood supply to the scaphoid influence healing?
    ➤ More proximal injuries have a higher rate of AVN

520. What physical exam findings are suspicious for a scaphoid fracture?
    ➤ Anatomic snuffbox tenderness
    ➤ Tenderness of the volar tuberosity

521. Which scaphoid fracture physical exam finding is most specific?
    ➤ Volar tuberosity tenderness

522. What is a humpback deformity?
    ➤ Apex dorsal deformity of a scaphoid fracture

523. What approach to the scaphoid is most commonly used for proximal pole fractures?
    ➤ Dorsal

524. What approach to the scaphoid is most commonly used for distal pole fractures and those with humpback deformities?
    ➤ Volar

525. What is a SNAC wrist?
    ➤ **S**caphoid **N**onunion **A**dvanced **C**ollapse

Hand

526. What are the radiographic stages of a SNAC wrist?
    - Stage I: Arthritis of scaphoid and radial styloid
    - Stage II: Stage I + Scaphocapitate arthritis
    - Stage III: Panscaphoid arthritis
527. What is a SLAC wrist?
    - **S**capho**L**unate **A**dvanced **C**ollapse
528. What is the SLAC wrist classification?
    - Watson Classification
        - Stage I: Arthritis of scaphoid and radial styloid
        - Stage II: Stage I + Scaphoid facet arthritis
        - Stage III: Stage II + Capitolunate arthritis
529. Which joint is commonly spared in a SLAC wrist?
    - Radiolunate
530. What deformity results from chronic scapholunate ligament injury?
    - DISI – **D**orsal **I**ntercalated **S**egment **I**nstability
531. Why does DISI occur following scapholunate ligament injury?
    - Coupled motion between the scaphoid and lunate is lost
        - The intact lunotriquetral ligament causes lunate extension
532. What does the Watson test evaluate?
    - Scapholunate instability
533. How is the Watson test performed?
    - Volar pressure over the distal scaphoid while the wrist is taken from ulnar to radial deviation
        - A "clunk" indicates instability

Hand

534. What is the eponym for atraumatic AVN of the scaphoid?
    ➢ Preiser's disease

Lunate

535. What is the classification for perilunate injuries?
    ➢ Mayfield Classification
        - Stage I: Scapholunate dissociation
        - Stage II: Stage I + Lunocapitate disruption
        - Stage III: Stage II + Lunotriquetral disruption
        - Stage IV: Lunate dislocation

536. What is the difference between lunate and perilunate dislocations?
    ➢ Lunate dislocation: The lunate is dislocated from the intact carpus
    ➢ Perilunate dislocation: The carpus dislocates while the lunate stays in its anatomic position

537. What deformity results from chronic lunotriquetral ligament injury?
    ➢ VISI – **V**olar **I**ntercalated **S**egment **I**nstability

538. Why does VISI occur following a lunotriquetral ligament injury?
    ➢ Coupled motion between the triquetrum and lunate is lost
        - The intact scapholunate ligament causes lunate flexion

539. What is the eponym for AVN of the lunate?
    ➢ Kienbock's disease

Hand

540. What is the classification for Kienbock's disease?
    - Lichtman Classification
        - Stage I: No changes on x-ray
        - Stage II: Sclerosis of the lunate on x-ray
        - Stage III: Lunate collapse
            - A: Without scaphoid rotation
            - B: With scaphoid rotation
        - Stage IV: Degeneration of adjacent joints

Metacarpal

541. What associated injury must be evaluated with a metacarpal base fracture?
    - Carpometacarpal (CMC) joint dislocation

542. What are the acceptable nonoperative tolerances for metacarpal shaft fractures?
    - Index and long fingers: 20° of angulation
    - Ring finger: 30° of angulation
    - Small finger: 40° of angulation

543. How much shortening and rotation may be accepted with a metacarpal shaft fracture?
    - Shortening: 2-5mm
    - Rotation: None

544. What are the acceptable nonoperative tolerances for metacarpal neck fractures?
    - Index and long fingers: 15° of angulation
    - Ring finger: 40° of angulation
    - Small finger: 60° of angulation

545. Hyperextension of the MCPJ may lead to avulsion of what structure?
    - Volar plate

Hand

546. Why is traction avoided during the reduction of an MCPJ dislocation?
> May lead to interposition of the volar plate creating an irreducible dislocation

547. In what position should the hand be splinted following a metacarpal fracture?
> Intrinsic plus position: Slight wrist extension with MCP joint flexion and IP joint extension

548. Why is the intrinsic plus position recommended for metacarpal fractures?
> Keeps tension on the collateral ligaments to help prevent stiffness

549. What is the eponym for a fifth metacarpal neck fracture?
> Boxer's fracture

550. What is the eponym for a fifth metacarpal base fracture?
> Baby Bennett

Thumb

551. What is the eponym for a simple intra-articular first metacarpal base fracture?
> Bennett fracture

552. What is the eponym for an intra-articular first metacarpal base fracture with multiple fracture lines?
> Rolando fracture

553. What are the primary deforming forces to a fracture at the base of the first metacarpal?
> Abductor pollicis longus (APL) – pulls shaft proximally and dorsally

Hand

> Adductor pollicis – pulls distal metacarpal shaft ulnar

554. What ligament allows the volar-ulnar fracture fragment to stay reduced in a thumb metacarpal base fracture?

> Volar beak ligament

555. What are the eponyms for a thumb ulnar collateral ligament (UCL) injury?

> Gamekeeper's thumb
> Skier's thumb

556. What is a Stener lesion?

> Adductor pollicis aponeurosis becomes interposed between the avulsed UCL and the thumb

557. Why are Stener lesions important to recognize?

> They're unlikely to heal without surgery

558. When evaluating thumb UCL injuries, what ligament(s) are being assessed with the thumb in full extension?

> Accessory and proper UCL ligaments

559. When evaluating thumb UCL injuries, what ligament(s) are being assessed with the thumb in 30° of flexion?

> Proper UCL ligament only

560. What ligament is torn with a thumb CMC joint dislocation?

> Dorsoradial ligament

561. What deformity of the thumb is analogous to a swan neck deformity?

> Duck bill deformity

Hand

Phalanx

562. How are the phalanges numbered?
    - Proximal phalanx – P1
    - Middle phalanx – P2
    - Distal phalanx – P3

563. What is the eponym for an extraarticular distal phalanx fracture?
    - Tuft fracture

564. What should also be evaluated with distal phalanx fractures?
    - Nailbed injuries

565. What is the typical deformity of a proximal phalanx fracture?
    - Apex volar

566. What forces create an apex volar deformity following a proximal phalanx fracture?
    - Proximal fragment: Interossei flex fragment
    - Distal fragment: Central slip extends fragment

567. Which finger is most commonly involved in high-pressure injection injuries?
    - Nondominant index finger

568. What deformity may occur following disruption of the central slip of the finger?
    - Boutonniere's deformity

569. What is a swan neck deformity?
    - PIPJ hyperextension with DIPJ flexion – caused by volar plate laxity

Hand

Trigger Finger

570. What is trigger finger?
    ➢ Stenosing tenosynovitis of the flexor tendon sheath
571. Which pulley is primarily involved with trigger finger?
    ➢ A1
572. Which structure may be injured with A1 pulley release of the thumb?
    ➢ Radial digital nerve – crosses surgical field

Flexor Tendon Injuries

573. What are the zones of flexor tendon injuries?
    ➢ Zone I: Distal to FDS insertion
    ➢ Zone II: Between FDS insertion and the distal palmar crease
    ➢ Zone III: Palm
    ➢ Zone IV: Carpal Tunnel
    ➢ Zone V: Proximal to the wrist crease
574. What is the wrist tenodesis effect?
    ➢ Extension of the wrist should cause finger flexion
    ➢ Flexion of the wrist should cause finger extension
575. What structure may prevent flexor tendon retraction following a laceration?
    ➢ Vinculum
576. What is the quadriga effect?
    ➢ Over-tightening of an FDP tendon will prevent full flexion of the uninjured digits

Hand

- Remember: FDP tendons share a common muscle belly in the forearm

577. Flexor tendon advancement of what distance may cause quadriga?
   ➢ >1cm

578. With end-to-end repair of tendons, what is the most important factor to increasing the strength of the repair?
   ➢ Increasing the number of sutures strands that cross the repair

579. What upper extremity autologous graft is commonly used for tendon reconstruction?
   ➢ Palmaris longus

580. What two early passive motion protocols are commonly used following flexor tendon repair?
   ➢ Duran protocol – patient assisted flexion
   ➢ Kleinert protocol – dynamic splint assisted flexion

581. What is a Jersey finger?
   ➢ Avulsion injury of the FDP tendon from the distal phalanx

582. What is the classification for Jersey fingers?
   ➢ Leddy and Packer Classification
     - Type I: FDP retraction to the palm
     - Type II: Retraction to PIPJ
     - Type III: Retraction to DIPJ
     - Type IV: "Double Avulsion" – Osseous avulsion from the distal phalanx with tendon avulsion from the osseous fragment
     - Type V: Comminuted bony avulsion

Hand

Extensor Tendon Injuries

583. What are the zones of extensor tendon injuries?
- Zone I: DIPJ and distal phalanx
- Zone II: Middle phalanx
- Zone III: PIPJ
- Zone IV: Proximal phalanx
- Zone V: MCPJ
- Zone VI: Metacarpal
- Zone VII: Radiocarpal joint
- Zone VIII: Distal forearm

584. In which zone is the extensor tendon most commonly injured?
- Zone VI – Metacarpal

585. What does the Elson test assess for?
- Integrity of the central slip

586. What is a Mallet finger?
- Disruption of the terminal extensor tendon on the distal phalanx

587. What is the classification for Mallet fingers?
- Doyle's Classification
  - Type I: Closed injury ± fracture
  - Type II: Open injury
  - Type III: Open injury with loss of tendon substance
  - Type IV: Fracture
    - A: Physeal injury
    - B: 20-30% articular surface involvement
    - C: >50% articular surface involvement

588. What is the name of the splint used to treat Mallet fingers?

Hand

- Stax splint

589. What are the surgical indications for repair of bony mallet injuries?
    - DIPJ subluxation
    - Bony avulsion involving >50% of the joint surface

Carpometacarpal Arthritis

590. What is the classification for CMC arthritis of the thumb?
    - Eaton and Littler Classification
        - Stage I: Widening of joint space, <1/3 subluxation
        - Stage II: Osteophytes <2mm, 1/3 subluxation
        - Stage III: Osteophytes >2mm, significant joint space narrowing, >1/3 subluxation
        - Stage IV: Erosion of scaphotrapezial joint

591. What physical exam finding is indicative of basilar thumb arthritis?
    - CMC grind test – pain with axial loading and circumduction

592. Successful surgical management of basilar thumb arthritis involves the removal of which bone?
    - Trapezium

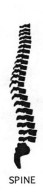
SPINE

Spine

General Anatomy

593. What are the normal values for cervical lordosis, thoracic kyphosis and lumbar lordosis?
   - ➢ Cervical lordosis: 15°
   - ➢ Thoracic kyphosis: 40°
   - ➢ Lumbar lordosis: 60°

594. What is the orientation of the superior facets in the cervical, thoracic and lumbar spines?
   - ➢ Cervical: **B**ack, **U**p, **M**edial
   - ➢ Thoracic: **B**ack, **U**p, **L**ateral
   - ➢ Lumbar: **B**ack, **M**edial
     - Remember: **BUM**, **BUL**, **BM**

595. What are the two parts of an intervertebral disc?
   - ➢ Annulus fibrosis and Nucleus pulposus

596. What type of collagen makes up the annulus fibrosis?
   - ➢ Type 1

597. What type of collagen makes up the nucleus pulposus?
   - ➢ Type 2

598. What are the three columns of the spine and what are their contents?
   - ➢ Anterior: Anterior longitudinal ligament (ALL), Anterior 2/3 of the vertebral body
   - ➢ Middle: Posterior longitudinal ligament (PLL), Posterior 1/3 of the vertebral body
   - ➢ Posterior: Posterior ligamentous complex (PLC), Spinous process, Lamina, Pedicles, Facets

Spine

599. What are the ascending sensory tracts and their functions?
    - Dorsal columns – deep touch, proprioception, and vibratory
    - Lateral spinothalamic – pain and temperature
    - Ventral columns – light touch

600. What is the name of the descending motor tract?
    - Lateral corticospinal tract

601. What is the main vascular supply to the descending motor tract?
    - Anterior spinal artery – supplies the anterior 2/3 of the spinal cord

602. What is the name of the anterior segmental artery that supplies the lower half of the spinal cord?
    - Artery of Adamkiewicz

603. What articulation in the cervical spine provides the majority of flexion and extension?
    - Occiput – C1, 50%

604. What articulation in the cervical spine provides the majority of rotation?
    - C1 – C2, 50%

605. What ligamentous structure maintains close contact between the atlas and odontoid?
    - Posterior transverse ligament

606. The posterior transverse ligament may be compromised in what patient population?
    - Rheumatoid arthritis
    - Excessively lax in patients with Down Syndrome

607. In the cervical spine, a paracentral or far lateral disc herniation affects which nerve root?

Spine

> - Exiting nerve root
>   - A paracentral or far lateral herniation at C4/5 affects C5

608. What vertebral level correlates with the hyoid cartilage, thyroid cartilage, cricoid cartilage, carotid tubercle, tip of the scapula, and iliac crest?

> - Hyoid cartilage: C3
> - Thyroid cartilage: C4-5
> - Cricoid cartilage: C6
> - Carotid tubercle: C6
> - Tip of the scapula: T7
> - Iliac crest: L4-5

609. At what level does the spinal cord end in adults?

> - L1

610. What is the term given to the tapered distal end of the spinal cord?

> - Conus medullaris

611. What is the relationship of the numbered nerve root to its associated pedicle in the cervical, thoracic and lumbar spines?

> - Cervical: Nerve root exits above the associated pedicle
>   - C4 nerve root exits above the C4 pedicle
> - Thoracic: Nerve root exits below the associated pedicle
>   - T4 nerve root exits below the T4 pedicle
> - Lumbar: Nerve root exits below the associated pedicle
>   - L4 nerve root exits below the L4 pedicle

Spine

612. Which pedicle has the narrowest diameter?
    ➢ T4
613. Which pedicle is the shortest in length?
    ➢ T4
614. In the lumbar spine, a paracentral disc herniation affects which nerve root?
    ➢ Traversing (lower) nerve root
        ▪ A paracentral herniation at L4/5 affects L5
615. In the lumbar spine, a far lateral disc herniation affects which nerve root?
    ➢ Exiting (upper) nerve root
        ▪ A far lateral herniation at L4/5 affects L4
616. What are the landmarks for pedicle screw placement in the thoracic and lumbar spines?
    ➢ Thoracic: Upper 1/3 of the transverse process and just lateral to a vertical line through the facet joint
    ➢ Lumbar: Middle of the transverse process and lateral border of the facet joint
617. What defines pelvic incidence?
    ➢ Pelvic tilt + Sacral slope

Spine

Trauma

Vertebral Fractures

618. What is a Hangman's fracture?
    - Traumatic spondylolisthesis of the axis (C2) following fractures to the bilateral lamina, pars or pedicles
619. What is a Clay-Shoveler's fracture?
    - Spinous process fracture in the lower cervical or upper thoracic spine
620. What is a burst fracture?
    - Vertebral body fracture involving the anterior and middle columns
621. What is a Chance fracture?
    - Flexion-distraction injury where the anterior column fails under compression and the posterior and middle columns fail under tension

Spinal Cord Injuries

622. What is the classification for spinal cord injuries?
    - ASIA (American Spinal Injury Association) Classification
        - A: Complete injury, No Motor, No Sensory
        - B: Incomplete injury, No Motor, Sensory preserved in sacral segments
        - C: Incomplete injury, Motor preserved, Strength <3/5
        - D: Incomplete injury, Motor preserved, Strength >3/5

- E: Incomplete injury, Motor and sensory function normal

623. What vital signs are indicative of spinal shock?
    - Bradycardia and hypotension
624. How long does spinal shock typically last?
    - 48 hours
625. What is the bulbocavernosus reflex?
    - Anal sphincter contraction following squeezing of the glans penis or pulling on foley catheter
626. What suggests resolution of spinal shock?
    - Return of the bulbocavernosus reflex or any reflexes distal to the injury
        - Bulbocavernosus reflex is typically the first to return
627. What aspect of a spinal cord injury cannot be completely evaluated until resolution of spinal shock?
    - Neurologic deficits
628. What is the most common incomplete spinal cord injury?
    - Central cord syndrome
629. What symptom pattern is suggestive of central cord syndrome?
    - Motor deficits that are worse in the upper extremities compared to the lower extremities
630. What injury mechanisms commonly result in central cord syndrome?
    - Extension type injuries
631. What is Brown-Sequard syndrome?
    - Hemi-transection of the spinal cord

Spine

632. What symptom pattern is suggestive of Brown-Sequard Syndrome?
    - ➢ Ipsilateral loss of motor function, proprioception and vibratory sensation
    - ➢ Contralateral loss of pain and temperature below the level of injury

633. What exam findings are suggestive of Cauda-Equina Syndrome?
    - ➢ Bowel and/or bladder dysfunction, saddle anesthesia, leg pain

634. What is the most common cause of Cauda-Equina Syndrome?
    - ➢ Massive central herniated disc, usually at L5-S1

635. What study may be performed to evaluate the spine in a patient who is unable to receive an MRI?
    - ➢ CT Myelogram

Spine

Spinal Conditions

Cervical Myelopathy

636. What is cervical myelopathy?
> ➤ Cervical spinal cord compression resulting in clumsiness of the hands and gait abnormalities

637. What upper extremity symptoms are commonly seen with cervical myelopathy?
> ➤ Hand clumsiness, positive Hoffman's sign, finger escape sign, sustained clonus, inverted radial reflex, hyperreflexia

638. What is the finger escape sign?
> ➤ When asked to hold the fingers extended and adducted, the small finger "escapes" into abduction due to intrinsic weakness

639. How is a Hoffman's test performed?
> ➤ Stabilize the middle phalanx of the long finger. Flick the distal phalanx into flexion allowing it to bounce back into extension. Reflexive flexion of the thumb IP joint indicates a positive test

Ankylosing Spondylitis (AS)

640. Which human leukocyte antigen (HLA) is highly associated with AS?
> ➤ HLA-B27

641. What radiographic findings are suggestive of AS?
> ➤ Vertebral scalloping "bamboo spine", marginal syndesmophytes

642. How do syndesmophytes differ from osteophytes?

Spine

> - Syndesmophytes are perpendicular to the vertebral body end plates
> - Osteophytes are parallel to the end plates

643. What additional study should be performed in a patient with AS and neck pain following trauma?

> - CT scan of the cervical spine to evaluate for fracture

Diffuse Idiopathic Skeletal Hyperostosis

644. How is Diffuse Idiopathic Skeletal Hyperostosis (DISH) defined?

> - Nonmarginal syndesmophytes involving 4 contiguous vertebrae

645. What characteristic radiographic finding is suggestive of DISH?

> - "Flowing candle wax" – diffuse calcification of the anterior longitudinal ligament

646. How does sacroiliac (SI) joint involvement differ between AS and DISH?

> - AS – bilateral sacroiliitis
> - DISH – no SI involvement

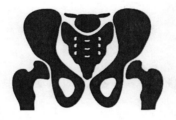

PELVIS

Pelvis

General Anatomy

647. What nerve root lies anterior to the sacral ala?
    ➢ L5
648. What artery crosses the SI joint anteriorly?
    ➢ Superior gluteal artery
649. Following pelvic ring injuries, is venous or arterial intrapelvic bleeding more common?
    ➢ Venous – 80%
650. If arterial bleeding does occur, what is the most common source?
    ➢ Superior gluteal artery
651. What muscles attach to the iliac crest?
    ➢ Tensor fascia latae, Gluteus medius, Iliacus, Latissimus dorsi, Abdominal muscles, Erector spinae muscles
652. What structures exit the greater sciatic notch above the piriformis?
    ➢ Superior gluteal vessels and nerve
653. What structures traverse the greater sciatic notch below the piriformis?
    ➢ Inferior gluteal vessels and nerve, Internal pudendal vessels, Pudendal nerve, Sciatic nerve, Posterior femoral cutaneous nerve, Nerve to obturator internus, Nerve to quadratus femoris
654. What structures traverse the lesser sciatic notch?
    ➢ Obturator internus tendon, Nerve to obturator internus, Pudendal nerve, Internal pudendal artery

Pelvis

655. What is the corona mortis?
> Vascular anastomosis between the **E**xternal **I**liac (Epigastric) and **O**bturator (Internal Iliac) vessels
  - Remember: Vowels – A,**E**,**I**,**O**,U

656. On average, the corona mortis is how far posterolateral to the pubic symphysis?
> 6.8cm

657. What are the windows of the ilioinguinal approach?
> Medial window: Medial to external iliac vessels
> Middle window: Between external iliac vessels and iliopsoas
> Lateral window: Lateral to iliopsoas

658. Through which window is the corona mortis encountered?
> Medial window

659. What is the most commonly injured structure during the ilioinguinal approach?
> Lateral femoral cutaneous nerve

660. What is the Space of Retzius?
> Space posterior to the pubic symphysis and anterior to the bladder

661. The sacrospinous ligaments resist what motion?
> External rotation

662. The sacrotuberous ligaments resist what motion?
> Vertical shear

663. Which ligament complex is most important for pelvic ring stability?
> Posterior sacroiliac complex

Pelvis

Trauma

Pelvic Ring

664. What are the two classification systems for pelvic ring injuries?
    - Young-Burgess Classification
    - Tile Classification
665. What is the Young-Burgess Classification?
    - Anterior Posterior Compression (APC)
        - APC I: ≤2.5cm pubic symphysis diastasis
        - APC II: >2.5cm pubic symphysis diastasis, sacrotuberous and sacrospinous ligaments disrupted, anterior SI ligaments disrupted
            - Posterior SI ligaments intact, rotationally unstable
        - APC III: APC II + Posterior SI ligament disruption
            - Rotationally and vertically unstable
    - Lateral Compression (LC)
        - LC I: Pubic symphysis fracture + SI compression fracture
        - LC II: LC I + Iliac wing fracture (Crescent fracture)
        - LC III: LC II + Contralateral APC III (Windswept pelvis)
    - Vertical Shear (VS)
666. What is the Tile Classification?
    - Tile Classification
        - A: Rotationally and vertically stable

Pelvis

- B: Rotationally unstable, vertically stable
- C: Rotationally and vertically unstable

667. What is the most common cause of death following an APC injury?

> Hemorrhage

668. What is the most common cause of death following an LC injury?

> Traumatic brain injury (TBI)

669. In the trauma bay, what is the initial treatment for a hemodynamically unstable patient with an APC pelvic injury?

> Apply a pelvic binder or sheet

670. Where should a pelvic binder or sheet be placed?

> Centered over the greater trochanters

671. How does the use of a pelvic binder or sheet help with hemodynamic instability?

> Decreases intrapelvic volume

672. Use of a pelvic binder or sheet is not indicated with which injuries?

> LC

673. In addition to a binder or sheet, what else may help to reduce intrapelvic volume?

> Internally rotating and taping the lower extremities together

674. Why does an APC pelvic injury look less severe on CT-imaging than on initial radiographs?

> Curve of the CT gantry under the patient internally rotates the hemipelvis

675. What is a Morel-Lavallee lesion?

> Closed, internal degloving injury

Pelvis

676. What is the eponym for an isolated iliac wing fracture that does not extend into the SI joint?
    ➤ Duverney fracture
677. What are the two most common pin site locations for placing a pelvic external fixator?
    ➤ Supra-acetabular and Iliac crest
678. What is the classification for sacrum fractures?
    ➤ Denis Classification
        - Zone 1: Fracture lateral to the foramina
        - Zone 2: Fracture through the foramina
        - Zone 3: Fracture medial to the foramina
679. Which sacral fracture has the highest rate of neurologic deficit?
    ➤ Denis Zone 3: Fractures medial to the foramina
680. What does a "U-type" sacral fracture represent?
    ➤ Spinopelvic dissociation

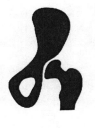

HIP

Hip

General Anatomy

681. What ligament crosses the inferior aspect of the acetabulum?
    - ➢ Transverse acetabular ligament
682. What is the normal neck-shaft angle of the proximal femur?
    - ➢ 130°
683. What is the primary blood supply to the femoral head in adults?
    - ➢ Lateral epiphyseal artery of the medial femoral circumflex artery
684. The hip center is most commonly at the same height as which other osseous structure?
    - ➢ Tip of the greater trochanter
685. What defines the 4 quadrants of the acetabulum for transacetabular screw placement?
    - ➢ A line drawn from the ASIS through the center of the acetabulum and a second line drawn perpendicular to the first at the center of the acetabulum
      - Posterior superior, Posterior inferior, Anterior superior, and Anterior inferior
686. What structures are at risk with screw placement into each quadrant of the acetabulum?
    - ➢ Posterior superior: Superior gluteal nerve and vessels, Sciatic nerve
      - This is considered the Safe Zone

Hip

- Posterior inferior: Inferior gluteal nerve, Internal pudendal artery
- Anterior superior: External iliac vessels
- Anterior inferior: Obturator vessels

687. What are the structures of the anterior column?
   - Anterior wall, Superior pubic ramus, Ilium

688. What are the structures of the posterior column?
   - Posterior wall, Ischial tuberosity, Sciatic notch, Quadrilateral surface

689. What is the most common relationship of the sciatic nerve to the piriformis tendon?
   - Sciatic nerve is anterior to piriformis tendon

690. What are the short external rotators of the hip?
   - Piriformis, Superior gamellus, Obturator internus, Inferior gamellus, Quadratus femoris

691. What position should the leg be placed in to decrease tension on the sciatic nerve?
   - Hip extension and knee flexion

692. What nerve must be identified and retracted during the anterior approach to the hip?
   - Lateral femoral cutaneous nerve

693. If the lateral femoral cutaneous nerve is injured, what is the resulting condition called?
   - Meralgia paresthetica

694. During the anterior approach to the hip, what vessels are encountered between the sartorius and tensor fascia latae?
   - Ascending branches of the lateral femoral circumflex vessels

Hip

695. What defines the subtrochanteric area of the femur?
    > ➤ Area between the lesser trochanter and 5cm distal

696. What are the deforming forces on a subtrochanteric femur fracture?
    > ➤ Proximal fragment: Abduction (Gluteus medius and minimus), Flexion (Iliopsoas), External rotation (Short external rotators)
    > ➤ Distal fragment: Adduction and Shortening (Adductors)

697. Where do the direct and indirect heads of the rectus femoris originate?
    > ➤ Direct head: Anterior inferior iliac spine
    > ➤ Indirect head: Supraacetabular ridge

698. Which nerve is at risk if the Gluteus medius is split more than 5cm proximal to the greater trochanter?
    > ➤ Superior gluteal nerve

699. Which vessel is at risk while dividing the quadratus femoris?
    > ➤ Medial femoral circumflex artery

700. Where does the hip capsule insert distally?
    > ➤ Anteriorly along the intertrochanteric crest
    > ➤ Posteriorly along the distal femoral neck

701. What muscle inserts on the lesser trochanter?
    > ➤ Iliopsoas

Trauma

Acetabulum

702. What is the classification for acetabulum fractures?
> - Letournel Classification
>   - Elementary fractures
>   - Posterior wall
>   - Anterior wall
>   - Posterior column
>   - Anterior column
>   - Transverse
>   - Associated fractures
>   - Both column
>   - Transverse-Posterior wall
>   - T-type
>   - Posterior column-Posterior wall
>   - Anterior column-Posterior hemi-transverse

703. Which elementary acetabulum fracture is the only one to involve both columns?
> - Transverse

704. What is the most common elementary acetabulum fracture?
> - Posterior wall

705. What is the most common associated acetabulum fracture?
> - Transverse posterior wall

706. Which acetabulum fracture is highly associated with posterior hip dislocations?
> - Posterior wall

Hip

707. Fractures involving what percentage of the posterior wall are highly associated with hip joint instability?
    ➤ ≥40%

708. What test can be performed to assess the stability of the hip joint following posterior wall fracture?
    ➤ Exam under anesthesia (EUA)

709. How can you measure the weight-bearing surface of the acetabulum on a fine cut (2mm) CT scan?
    ➤ Superior 10mm (5 cuts) of the acetabulum on axial views

710. What are the 5 most common approaches used to fix acetabular fractures?
    ➤ Ilioinguinal, Iliofemoral, Modified Stoppa, Kocher-Langenbach, and Extended iliofemoral

711. Which approach is associated with the highest risk of heterotopic ossification?
    ➤ Extended iliofemoral

712. What is the most common complication following acetabulum fractures?
    ➤ Post-traumatic arthritis

713. Postoperatively, what type of weight-bearing has the lowest joint reactive forces?
    ➤ Touch-down weight-bearing

714. What is the difference between a posterior approach for ORIF of the acetabulum and the posterior approach for a THA?
    ➤ Must protect the medial femoral circumflex artery with ORIF

- Do not transect quadratus femoris muscle or take the short external rotators directly off bone (leave 1cm cuff) when performing ORIF

Hip Dislocations

715. How will the lower extremity appear with a posterior hip dislocation?
    ➢ Shortened, adducted, and internally rotated
        ▪ Rotation may not be present if there is a large displaced posterior wall fracture

716. How will the lower extremity appear with an anterior hip dislocation?
    ➢ Abducted and externally rotated

717. What is the difference between a complex and a simple hip dislocation?
    ➢ Simple: Dislocation without associated fracture
    ➢ Complex: Dislocation with associated acetabulum or proximal femur fracture

718. What knee injury should you specifically evaluate for in a patient with a posterior hip dislocation following a motor vehicle crash?
    ➢ PCL injury secondary to impaction with the dashboard

719. Which nerve is most commonly injured following a posterior hip dislocation?
    ➢ Sciatic nerve
        ▪ Most commonly the peroneal division

720. The incidence of what complication increases with increased time to reduction of a dislocated hip?
    ➢ Femoral head AVN

Hip

721. Following successful reduction of a hip dislocation what type of immobilization should be used?
    ➤ Knee immobilizer and abduction pillow

722. What imaging should be obtained following a native hip reduction?
    ➤ CT scan to evaluate the reduction, marginal impaction, loose bodies in the joint, and associated acetabular and femoral head fractures

723. What may be done in an unstable posterior hip dislocation to help keep the hip reduced prior to surgery?
    ➤ Skeletal traction

Femoral Head & Neck

724. What is the classification for femoral head fractures?
    ➤ Pipkin Classification
        - Type I: Infrafoveal fracture
        - Type II: Suprafoveal fracture
        - Type III: Type I or II with associated femoral neck fracture
        - Type IV: Type I or II with associated acetabulum fracture

725. What are the operative indications for femoral head fractures?
    ➤ Intra-articular loose body, Pipkin II with >1mm step-off, Pipkin III & IV fractures

726. Which surgical approach allows for improved visualization of the femoral head during ORIF?
    ➤ Anterior or anterolateral

Hip

- Posterior approach has the worse visualization and is associated with poorer outcomes

727. What is the most common treatment for femoral head fractures in elderly patients?
    - Arthroplasty

728. What are the two classifications for femoral neck fractures?
    - Garden Classification – based on displacement
        - Type I: Incomplete, non-displaced fracture
            - Valgus impacted
        - Type II: Complete, non-displaced fracture
        - Type III: Complete fracture with <100% displacement
        - Type IV: Complete fracture with >100% displacement
    - Pauwel's Classification – based the trajectory of the fracture line from the horizontal plane
        - Type I: <30° angle
        - Type II: 30-50° angle
        - Type III: >50° angle

729. How are femoral neck fractures described by anatomic location?
    - Subcapital, transcervical, and basicervical

730. How will the lower extremity appear with a hip fracture?
    - Shortened and externally rotated

731. What are three most common surgical treatment options for femoral neck fractures?
    - ORIF, hemiarthroplasty, and total hip arthroplasty

Hip

732. In a young patient with a femoral neck fracture, what is the treatment of choice?
   ➢ ORIF
      ▪ Dynamic hip screw (DHS) or 3 screws

733. What is the preferred screw configuration when treating with 3 screws?
   ➢ Inverted triangle

734. In which order are the screws placed when utilizing an inverted triangle configuration?
   ➢ First: Inferiorly along the calcar
   ➢ Second: Posterior-superior
   ➢ Third: Anterior-superior

735. What complication may occur with screw placement starting distal to the lesser trochanter?
   ➢ Subtrochanteric fracture secondary to creation of a stress riser

736. What are the two types of femoral neck stress fractures?
   ➢ Compression sided (inferior)
   ➢ Tension sided (superior)

737. Which femoral neck stress fracture may be treated nonoperatively?
   ➢ Compression sided

Intertrochanteric Fractures

738. How does the healing potential of intertrochanteric (IT) fractures differ from femoral neck fractures?

Hip

- IT fractures are extracapsular and have a better healing potential due to their periosteum and soft tissue attachments

739. What makes an IT fracture unstable?
    - Reverse obliquity
    - Fracture extension into the subtrochanteric region
    - Disrupted medial calcar
    - Disruption of the lateral cortex

740. What are the non-arthroplasty surgical treatment options for IT fractures?
    - Sliding hip screw (SHS), cephalomedullary nail (CMN)

741. Sliding hip screws should be avoided in which type of IT fractures?
    - Unstable fracture patterns

742. What is the Tip-to-Apex distance (TAD)?
    - Combined distance from the tip of the screw to the apex of the femoral head on the AP and lateral views

743. What is the importance of the TAD?
    - TAD >25mm is associated with screw cutout

Subtrochanteric Fractures

744. What is the classification for subtrochanteric femur fractures?
    - Russel-Taylor Classification
      - Type I: Intact piriformis fossa
        - IA: Lesser trochanter attached to the proximal fragment

- IB: Lesser trochanter detached from the proximal fragment
  - Type II: Fracture extends into the piriformis fossa
    - IIA: Stable posteromedial buttress
    - IIB: Comminution of the lesser trochanter

745. What features are suggestive of an atypical femur fracture?
  ➤ Subtrochanteric, absence of major trauma, transverse, lateral cortical thickening, medial cortical spike, prodromal symptoms, no comminution

746. What is the most common surgical treatment for subtrochanteric femur fractures?
  ➤ Intramedullary nail

747. What is the advantage of placing an IMN with the patient in the lateral decubitus position?
  ➤ Allows for easier reduction of fracture fragments

748. What is the most common malunion following antegrade IMN for subtrochanteric femur fractures?
  ➤ Varus and procurvatum

Sports

Femoroacetabular Impingement (FAI)

749. What is a Cam lesion?
    ➢ Aspherical femoral head
750. What is a Pincer lesion?
    ➢ Overhang of the anterosuperior acetabular rim
751. Cam lesions are most commonly seen in what patient population?
    ➢ Young athletic males
752. Pincer lesions are most commonly seen in what patient population?
    ➢ Middle aged females
753. What motion is most limited with FAI?
    ➢ Flexion, adduction, and internal rotation
754. Labral tears in which location are most common with FAI?
    ➢ Anterosuperior
755. In the treatment of FAI with hip arthroscopy, what nerve injury most commonly occurs secondary to traction?
    ➢ Pudendal nerve neuropraxia

Coxa Sultans (Snapping Hip)

756. What is the cause of internal coxa sultan?
    ➢ Iliopsoas tendon "snapping" over the femoral head or lesser trochanter
757. What is the cause of external coxa sultan?
    ➢ IT band "snapping" over the greater trochanter

Hip

758. What is the cause of intra-articular coxa sultan?
    ➢ Loose body within the hip joint

Hip

Adult Reconstruction

Total Hip Arthroplasty (THA)

759. What are the four most commonly used approaches for THA?
    - Anterior (Smith-Petersen)
    - Anterolateral (Watson-Jones)
    - Direct lateral (Hardinge)
    - Posterior (Southern-Moore)

760. What are the superficial and deep intervals for the anterior approach (Smith-Petersen) to the hip?
    - Superficial: Tensor fascia latae (Superior gluteal nerve) and Sartorius (Femoral nerve)
    - Deep: Gluteus medius (Superior gluteal nerve) and Rectus femoris (Femoral nerve)

761. What is the interval for the anterolateral approach (Watson-Jones) to the hip?
    - Tensor fascia latae (Superior gluteal nerve) and Gluteus medius (Superior gluteal nerve)

762. What is the posterior (Southern-Moore) approach to the hip?
    - Split Gluteus maximus (Inferior gluteal nerve). Retract Gluteus medius anteriorly. Identify Piriformis and short external rotators. Detach the Piriformis, Superior gamellus, Obturator internus, and Inferior gamellus from bone. Dislocate the hip

Hip

763. What is the classification for proximal femur bone quality?
> ➤ Dorr Classification
>   - Type A: Narrow canal with good bone
>   - "Champagne flute"
>   - Type B: Cortex narrowing with canal widening
>   - Type C: Thin cortex with wide canal
>   - "Stovepipe"

764. What type of femoral fixation is usually recommended for Dorr Type C femurs?
> ➤ Cemented femoral components

765. The acetabular cup should be placed with how much lateral inclination?
> ➤ 35-40°

766. The acetabular cup should be placed with how much anteversion?
> ➤ 20-30°
>   - Too much anteversion may cause impingement on the iliopsoas anteriorly

767. What soft tissue structure may be used to judge the position of the acetabular cup?
> ➤ Transverse acetabular ligament (TAL)

768. In what quadrant of the acetabulum can screws be placed most safely?
> ➤ Posterior-superior

769. When evaluating an AP pelvis radiograph, where should the acetabular cup be positioned relative to the radiographic lines of the pelvis?
> ➤ Medialized to the ilioischial line

Hip

> Inferior border of the cup aligned with the inferior border of the teardrop

770. The femoral component should be placed with how much anteversion?

> 15°

771. If a femoral stem is put in with too much anteversion, how will the patient's foot be position?

> In-toeing

772. What is femoral head offset?

> The distance from the center of the femoral head to the lateral greater trochanter

773. Excessively increased femoral head offset can lead to what complication?

> Trochanteric bursitis

774. How does increasing the head to neck ratio influence motion and stability?

> Increases motion and stability

775. What are the two fixation techniques for femoral stems?

> Cemented
> Press-fit

776. What is the difference between on-growth and in-growth press fit prostheses?

> In-growth: Porous coated – bone grows into the implant
> On-growth: Grit blasted – bone grows onto the implant

777. If a femur fracture is encountered during implant insertion what should be done?

Hip

> ➤ Removal of the implant, placement of cerclage wires, reimplantation

778. What radiographic factors demonstrate a well-fixed femoral component?
   ➤ Stress shielding around the proximal femur
   ➤ Regional calcar resorption (round off)
   ➤ New bone formation along the stem
     - "Spot welding"
   ➤ No subsidence of the stem

779. What symptoms suggest a loose femoral component?
   ➤ Thigh pain, start-up pain with walking

780. What are the most common bearing combinations for THA?
   ➤ Ceramic on polyethylene
   ➤ Ceramic on ceramic
   ➤ Metal (Cobalt-Chrome) on polyethylene

781. What combination has the best wear properties?
   ➤ Ceramic on ceramic

782. Squeaking can be seen with which bearing surface?
   ➤ Ceramic on ceramic

783. Pseudotumors are a complication seen with which bearing combination?
   ➤ Metal on metal

784. What complication is more common utilizing a posterior (Southern-Moore) approach?
   ➤ Dislocation

785. What intraoperative complication is more common utilizing an anterior (Smith-Petersen) approach?

- Femur fracture

786. What complication is more common following utilization of an anterolateral (Watson-Jones) approach?
    - Limping secondary to weak abductors
        - Trendelenburg gait

787. What is the classification for hip periprosthetic fractures?
    - Vancouver Classification
        - Type A: Peritrochanteric fractures
            - A_G: Greater trochanter fracture
            - A_L: Lesser trochanter fracture
        - Type B: Fracture around or just distal to the stem
            - B1: Stable stem, Good bone stock
            - B2: Loose stem, Good bone stock
            - B3: Loose stem, Poor bone stock
        - Type C: Fracture well distal to the stem

788. When treating a periprosthetic fracture, fixation must bypass the fracture site by what distance?
    - 2 cortical diameters

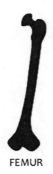
FEMUR

Femur

General Anatomy

789. What muscles are in the anterior compartment of the thigh?
   ➢ Sartorius, Rectus femoris, Vastus lateralis, Vastus intermedius, and Vastus medialis

790. What muscles are in the posterior compartment of the thigh?
   ➢ Biceps femoris, Semimembranosus, and Semitendinosus

791. What muscles are in the medial compartment of the thigh?
   ➢ Gracilis, Adductors longus, Adductor brevis, and Adductor magnus

792. What is the name for the crest of bone along the posterior middle third of the femur?
   ➢ Linea aspera

793. In which direction does the femur bow?
   ➢ Anteriorly

794. What is the isthmus of the femur?
   ➢ Narrowest part of the femoral canal – juncture of the proximal and middle thirds

795. What shape is the distal femur in the axial plane?
   ➢ Trapezoidal

796. What muscle from the lower leg originates on the distal femur?
   ➢ Gastrocnemius

797. What is the only muscle of the thigh that is innervated by the peroneal division of the sciatic nerve?
   ➢ Short head of the biceps femoris

Trauma

Femoral Shaft

798. What is the classification for femoral shaft fractures?
    - Winquist Classification
        - Type 0: No comminution
        - Type I: Minimal comminution
        - Type II: >50% cortical contact
        - Type III: <50% cortical contact
        - Type IV: Segmental femur fracture with no cortical contact

799. The thigh can hold how much blood following a femoral shaft fracture?
    - 1-1.5L

800. In which direction should a distal femoral traction pin be placed?
    - Medial to lateral

801. Why is a distal femoral traction pin placed medial to lateral?
    - To avoid injury to the femoral artery

802. Where should a distal femoral traction pin be placed?
    - At the level of the proximal pole of the patella and centered on the femur in the sagittal plane

803. Where else may a traction pin be placed for femur fractures?
    - Proximal tibia

804. In which direction should a proximal tibial traction pin be placed?

Femur

> Lateral to medial

805. Why is a proximal tibial traction pin placed lateral to medial?

> To avoid injury to the common peroneal nerve

806. Where should a proximal tibial traction pin be placed?

> 2cm distal and 2cm posterior to tibial tubercle

807. What additional injury must be ruled out in a patient with a femoral shaft fracture?

> Ipsilateral femoral neck fracture

808. Femoral neck fractures associated with femoral shaft fractures have what characteristics?

> High Pauwel's angle (vertical)
> Basicervical
> Nondisplaced

809. What are the surgical treatment options for patients with ipsilateral femoral neck and shaft fractures?

> Retrograde intramedullary nail (IMN) with sliding hip screw or 3 screws

810. Which fracture receives priority in a patient with a femoral shaft and ipsilateral femoral neck fracture?

> Femoral neck

811. Why does the femoral neck fracture receive treatment priority?

> Risk of AVN

812. What four imaging modalities should be performed to rule out an ipsilateral femoral neck fracture in a patient with a femoral shaft fracture?

> AP internal rotation x-ray

> CT scan
> Intraoperative lateral fluoroscopy prior to fixation
> Postoperative AP and lateral hip x-rays

813. What are the two most common starting points for an antegrade IMN?
> Trochanteric and Piriformis fossa

814. What is the benefit of using a piriformis IMN?
> Starting point is in line with the femoral shaft

815. In which patients is it more difficult to use a piriformis IMN?
> Obese patients

816. What are indications for use of a retrograde IMN?
> Obesity
> Bilateral femur fractures
> Floating knee
> Distal femoral shaft fracture
> Ipsilateral femoral neck or acetabular fracture

817. What is the starting point for a retrograde IMN on the AP radiograph?
> Center of the intercondylar notch

818. What is the starting point of a retrograde IMN on the lateral radiograph?
> Anterior edge of Blumensaat's line

819. What structure is at risk with a starting point posterior to Blumensaat's line?
> ACL

820. What structures are at risk with the proximal AP screw in a retrograde femoral IMN?
> Femoral nerve and artery

Femur

Distal Femur

821. What deformity commonly occurs with distal femur fractures?
   ➢ Varus and extension

822. What are the deforming forces that lead to the varus and extension deformity?
   ➢ Extension – Gastrocnemius
   ➢ Varus – Adductor magnus

823. What is the name of a distal femur fracture that occurs in the coronal plane?
   ➢ Hoffa fracture

824. What percentage of distal femur fractures have a Hoffa fracture?
   ➢ 38%

825. Are Hoffa fractures more common medial or lateral?
   ➢ Lateral

826. With ORIF of the distal femur, what deformity may occur if a lateral femoral plate is placed too posteriorly?
   ➢ Medialization of the articular block
     - Referred to as a "golf club" or "hockey stick" deformity

827. What additional treatment option is available for patients with a non-reconstructable distal femur fracture?
   ➢ Distal femoral replacement

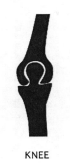

KNEE

Knee

General Anatomy

828. What is the largest sesamoid bone in the body?
    > Patella

829. The predominant blood supply to the patella enters the bone from which anatomic direction?
    > Inferomedial patella

830. Which patellar facet is larger?
    > Lateral

831. A Baker's cyst most commonly occurs between which two muscles?
    > Medial head of the Gastrocnemius and Semimembranosus

832. Which meniscus is "C-shaped" and which is circular?
    > Medial meniscus: "C-shaped"
    > Lateral meniscus: Circular

833. What are the vascular zones of the meniscus from peripheral to central?
    > Red-Red, Red-White, White-White

834. Which group of ligaments connect the meniscus to the tibial plateau?
    > Coronary ligaments

835. Which group of ligaments connect the lateral meniscus to the PCL?
    > Meniscofemoral ligaments

836. What are the two meniscofemoral ligaments?
    > Ligament of Humphrey and Ligament of Wrisberg

Knee

837. What is the relationship of the meniscofemoral ligaments to the PCL?
> - Ligament of Humphrey – anterior to the PCL
> - Ligament of Wrisberg – posterior to the PCL

838. What is the primary restraint to anterior translation in an ACL-deficient knee?
> - Posterior horn of the medial meniscus

839. What are the bundles of the ACL?
> - Anteromedial and Posterolateral

840. What bony landmark separates the bundles of the ACL?
> - Bifurcate ridge

841. What anatomic structure is referred to as "Resident's Ridge"?
> - Intercondylar ridge

842. What is the primary blood supply to the ACL?
> - Middle geniculate artery

843. What is the name of the tissue seen directly anterior to the ACL on arthroscopy?
> - Ligamentum mucosum

844. What are the bundles of the PCL?
> - Anterolateral and posteromedial

845. Is the medial or lateral tibial plateau more distal?
> - Medial tibial plateau

846. Is the medial or lateral tibial plateau more concave?
> - Medial tibial plateau

847. From proximal to distal, what tendons make up the pes anserine?
> - **S**artorius, **G**racilis, Semi**T**endinosus

Knee

- Remember: "**S**ay **G**race before **T**ea"

848. What are the layers of the lateral knee?
  - Layer 1: IT band, Biceps femoris
  - Layer 2: Patella retinaculum, Patellofemoral ligament
  - Layer 3:
    - Superficial: LCL, Fabellofibular ligament, Anterior lateral ligament
    - Deep: Arcuate ligament, Coronary ligament, Popliteus tendon, Popliteofibular ligament

849. What structure runs between layers 1 and 2 on the lateral knee?
  - Common peroneal nerve

850. What structure runs between the superficial and deep portions of layer 3 on the lateral knee?
  - Lateral geniculate artery

851. What tendon is visualized intraarticularly in the lateral knee?
  - Popliteus

852. What is the function of the popliteus muscle?
  - Internally rotates the tibia

853. What is the relationship between the origins of the LCL and the popliteus on the distal femur?
  - Popliteus originates anterior and distal to the LCL

854. What are the three main stabilizers of the posterolateral corner?
  - LCL, Popliteus tendon, Popliteofibular ligament

855. What three structures attach to the fibular head?

Knee

> From anterior to posterior: LCL, Popliteofibular ligament, Biceps femoris

856. What are the layers of the medial knee?
> Layer 1: Sartorius, Patellar retinaculum
> Layer 2: Semimembranosus, Superficial MCL, Medial Patellofemoral Ligament (MPFL), Posterior oblique ligament
> Layer 3: Deep MCL, Coronary ligaments

857. What structures run between layers 1 and 2 on the medial knee?
> Gracilis, Semitendinosus, and Saphenous nerve

858. What is the primary restraint to valgus stress of the knee?
> Superficial MCL

859. What is a bipartite patella?
> Failure of the superolateral corner of the patella to fuse

860. What muscle is deep to the vastus intermedius and is commonly encountered during anterior femoral exposure for TKA?
> Articularis genus

861. What is the function of the articularis genus muscle?
> Pulls the suprapatellar bursa superiorly with knee extension

862. The popliteal artery is located most closely to bone on which side of the knee?
> Laterally

863. Where are the medial and lateral geniculate arteries located?

Knee

- Medial geniculate: Medial tibial metaphysis
- Lateral geniculate: Just lateral to the lateral meniscus
  - Main source of bleeding with deep resection of the lateral meniscus

864. When removing the medial meniscus, what structure may be injured with too deep of a resection?

- Superficial MCL

865. Which four muscles make up the quadriceps tendon?

- Rectus femoris, Vastus lateralis, Vastus medialis, and Vastus intermedius

866. What is the innervation of the quadricep muscles?

- Femoral nerve

867. Numbness on the distal lateral portion of the knee following TKA is caused by injury to what cutaneous nerve?

- Infrapatellar branch of the saphenous nerve
  - Most common postoperative neuroma following TKA

Knee

Trauma

Patella

868. What surgical fixation methods may be used to treat patella fractures?
    ➤ Suture tension banding, K-wires, cerclage wires, plate and screws, screws alone

869. Which treatment option may be considered in distal or proximal pole fractures?
    ➤ Partial patellectomy

870. What fracture pattern is typically amenable to nonoperative management?
    ➤ Vertical fractures

871. What must remain intact in order to treat a patella fracture nonoperatively?
    ➤ Extensor mechanism

872. What structure may allow for the ability to perform a straight leg raise despite a patella fracture?
    ➤ Intact patellar retinaculum

873. If a complete patellectomy is performed, how much quadriceps strength is lost?
    ➤ 50%

Knee Dislocations

874. What is the classification for knee dislocations?
    ➤ Schneck Classification
        - KD I: (1 ligament) ACL or PCL disruption
        - KD II: (2 ligaments) ACL and PCL disruption

Knee

- KD III: (3 ligaments) ACL, PCL and Posteromedial corner (PMC) or Posterolateral corner (PLC) disruption
    - KD III-M: ACL, PCL, PLC, MCL disruption
    - KD III-L: ACL PCL, PLC, LCL disruption
- KD IV: (4 ligaments) ACL, PCL, PMC, PLC disruption
- KD V: Multi-ligamentous knee injury with periarticular fracture

875. Knee dislocations occur most commonly in which direction?
➢ Tibia anterior

876. What percentage of knee dislocations reduce spontaneously in the field?
➢ 50%

877. What associated injury must be evaluated immediately following reduction?
➢ Popliteal artery injury

878. What percentage of knee dislocations have an associated popliteal artery injury?
➢ 20-40%

879. Why is the popliteal artery susceptible to injury following knee dislocations?
➢ Tethered proximally at the popliteal hiatus and distally as the soleus arch

880. What type of popliteal artery injury is associated with an anterior dislocation?
➢ Intimal tear

Knee

881. What type of popliteal artery injury is associated with a posterior dislocation?
    ➢ Transection
882. Which nerve is most commonly injured with a knee dislocation?
    ➢ Common peroneal nerve
883. What is a Dimple Sign?
    ➢ Dimpling of the skin secondary to button-holing of the medial femoral condyle through the medial joint capsule
        ▪ This suggests an irreducible knee dislocation

Tibial Plateau

884. What is the classification for tibial plateau fractures?
    ➢ Schatzker Classification
        ▪ Type I: Lateral split
        ▪ Type II: Lateral split with depression
        ▪ Type III: Lateral depression only
        ▪ Type IV: Medial split
        ▪ Type V: Bicondylar
        ▪ Type VI: Metaphyseal-diaphyseal dissociation
885. What alternative classification may be used for tibial plateau fractures?
    ➢ Hohl and Moore Classification
        ▪ Type I: Coronal split
        ▪ Type II: Entire condyle
        ▪ Type III: Lateral plateau rim avulsion
        ▪ Type IV: Rim compression
        ▪ Type V: 4-part fractures

Knee

886. What intraarticular injury commonly occurs with a Schatzker Type II tibial plateau fracture?
    ➢ Lateral meniscus tear

887. Which Schatzker classification is said to be a "knee dislocation" equivalent?
    ➢ Type IV

888. With a Schatzker Type IV tibial plateau fracture, you should have a high suspicion for injury to which structure?
    ➢ Popliteal artery

889. If a difference in palpable pulse strength is noted, what test should be performed?
    ➢ Ankle Brachial Index (Normal is >0.9)

890. Which types of tibial plateau fractures have a high association with compartment syndrome?
    ➢ Schatzker Type V & VI

891. What are the operative indications for a tibial plateau fracture?
    ➢ Articular step-off >3mm
        ▪ Controversial – similar clinical outcomes with nonoperative management are seen with up to 8mm of step-off
    ➢ Condylar widening >5mm
    ➢ All bicondylar and medial plateau fractures
    ➢ Open fractures
    ➢ Varus/valgus instability

892. In a tibial plateau fracture requiring external fixation, should a CT scan be performed before or after fixator application?

> After - this allows for better surgical planning once the fracture is pulled out to length due to ligamentotaxis

893. During ORIF, what is commonly used to fill a metaphyseal void?

> Calcium phosphate – has the highest compressive strength of all substitutes

894. What substitute has a high rate of subsidence and drainage if used to fill a metaphyseal void?

> Calcium sulfate

895. Restoration of which factors are critical following ORIF of tibial plateau fractures?

> Length, mechanical alignment, and rotation

896. What is the most common complication following tibial plateau fractures?

> Post-traumatic arthritis

Knee

Sports

Anterior Cruciate Ligament (ACL)

897. Are males or females more susceptible to ACL tears?
   - Females

898. What are some of the theories as to why ACL injuries are more common in females?
   - Altered landing biomechanics
   - Increased valgus alignment of the knee
   - Narrower femoral notch
   - Differing hormone receptors and sequence of neuromuscular firing

899. What subjective history suggests an ACL injury?
   - Non-contact twisting mechanism
   - Audible "pop"
   - Immediate swelling
     - Hemarthrosis

900. What are the three physical exam tests for diagnosing ACL ruptures?
   - Anterior drawer, Lachman's, and Pivot shift

901. How is a pivot shift performed?
   - With a constant valgus and internal rotation force, the leg is moved from extension to flexion
     - Positive with reduction of the tibia, typically occurring around 30° of flexion

902. What is the most sensitive physical exam test for an ACL rupture?
   - Lachman's

Knee

903. What is the most specific physical exam test for an ACL rupture?
    ➤ Pivot shift

904. The anterior drawer primarily tests which ACL bundle?
    ➤ Anteromedial

905. The pivot shift primarily tests which bundle of the ACL?
    ➤ Posterolateral

906. A Segond fracture occurs following avulsion of which ligament?
    ➤ Anterolateral ligament (ALL)
        - Seen as an avulsion fracture of the proximal lateral aspect of the tibia and is pathognomonic for an ACL tear

907. What is the typical pattern of bone bruising seen on MRI following an ACL tear?
    ➤ Anterior or middle 1/3 of the lateral femoral condyle and posterior 1/3 of the lateral tibial plateau

908. Are medial or lateral meniscus tears more common with acute ACL injuries?
    ➤ Lateral

909. What are the two most commonly used grafts for ACL reconstruction?
    ➤ Bone-Patellar Tendon-Bone (BTB)
    ➤ Quadruple hamstring (Gracilis and Semitendinosus)

910. What is the benefit of using a BTB graft?
    ➤ Bone to bone healing

Knee

911. What is the drawback of using a BTB graft?
    ➢ Increased anterior knee pain
912. What is the benefit of using a quadrable hamstring graft?
    ➢ Graft has the highest load to failure
913. What are the drawbacks of using a quadrable hamstring graft?
    ➢ Theoretical risk of hamstring weakness with autograft, stretching of the graft, tunnel widening, and slower healing
914. What is the most common cause of ACL reconstruction failure?
    ➢ Tunnel malpositioning
915. How is the femoral tunnel most commonly malpositioned?
    ➢ Too vertical
916. Where should the femoral tunnel be positioned?
    ➢ 9-10 O'clock position and 6-8mm from posterior cortex (leaves 1-2mm of cortical margin)
917. What landmarks may be used for placement of the tibial tunnel?
    ➢ 1cm anterior to the PCL
    ➢ Slightly anterior to the medial tibial eminence
    ➢ In line with the posterior border of the anterior horn of the lateral meniscus
918. The knee should be held in what position when tensioning the graft?
    ➢ Approximately 20° of flexion with a reverse Lachman motion

- The all inside technique tensions the graft with the knee in full extension

919. What complication occurs if the tibial tunnel is positioned too anteriorly?
   ➢ Graft impingement in extension

920. What complication occurs if the tibial tunnel is positioned too posteriorly?
   ➢ Graft impingement with the PCL

921. What complication occurs if the femoral tunnel is positioned too anteriorly?
   ➢ Knee will be tight in flexion and loose in extension

922. What complication occurs if the femoral tunnel is positioned too posteriorly?
   ➢ Knee will be loose in flexion and tight in extension

923. What is a cyclops lesion?
   ➢ Localized fibrosis of the native ACL stump following reconstruction

924. What commonly associated injury, if missed, may compromise ACL reconstruction?
   ➢ Posterolateral corner injury
      - These should be repaired simultaneously or staged with the PLC reconstruction performed first

Collateral Ligaments (MCL, LCL)

925. How are collateral ligament injuries graded?
   ➢ Grade I: Stretch injury
   ➢ Grade II: Partial tear

Knee

> Grade III: Complete tear

926. What is the eponym for a calcified MCL?
   > Pellegrini-Stieda lesion

927. What does the presence of a Pellegrini-Stieda lesion suggest?
   > Chronic MCL injury or insufficiency

928. Where do MCL injuries typically occur?
   > Femoral origin

929. When explicitly testing the integrity of the MCL or LCL, the knee should be held in what position?
   > 30° of flexion

930. What does varus or valgus laxity in full extension suggest?
   > Combined collateral and cruciate and/or capsular injury

931. What does the dial test assess?
   > Posterolateral corner (PLC) injury

932. How do you perform the dial test?
   > Place the patient prone and externally rotate the tibia at both 90° and 30° of knee flexion and compare to the contralateral side

933. Asymmetry of >10° with the dial test at 30° of flexion indicates what?
   > Isolated PLC injury

934. Asymmetry of >10° with the dial test at both 30° and 90° of flexion indicates what?
   > Combined PLC and PCL injury

Knee

Meniscus Injuries

935. Are medial or lateral meniscus tears more common?
    - **M**edial
        - Remember: **M**edial = **M**ost Common
936. What symptoms are suggestive of a meniscus tear?
    - Mechanical symptoms (locking, clicking, catching, popping)
937. What is the most sensitive physical exam finding for a meniscus tear?
    - Joint line tenderness
938. What are provocative tests for assessing a meniscus tear?
    - McMurray's, Apley's, and Thessaly's test
939. What are common meniscus tear patterns?
    - Longitudinal, Radial, Bucket Handle, Parrot beak, and Complex
940. How does a meniscus tear appear on MRI?
    - Increased T2 signal within the meniscus that extends to the periphery
941. What is a "Double PCL" sign?
    - Bucket handle meniscus tear that flips into the notch and appears anterior and inferior to the native PCL on sagittal MRI
942. What is the treatment of choice for a degenerative meniscus tear?
    - Partial meniscectomy
943. Which meniscus tears are amendable to repair?
    - Tears within 3mm of the periphery (Red-Red zone) that are not degenerative

Knee

Discoid Meniscus

944. What is a discoid meniscus?
   ➢ Anatomical variant of a thicker and fuller crescent-shaped meniscus

945. What is the classification for a discoid meniscus?
   ➢ Watanabe Classification
     - Type I: Incomplete
     - Type II: Complete
     - Type III: Wrisberg variant – no posterior meniscotibial attachments

946. Is a discoid meniscus more common medially or laterally?
   ➢ Laterally

947. What x-ray findings may be indicative of a discoid meniscus?
   ➢ Increased joint space, flattening of the femoral condyle, and cupping of the tibial plateau

948. What MRI finding is consistent with a discoid meniscus?
   ➢ "Bow-tie sign" – 3 consecutive sagittal MRI cuts showing contiguous anterior and posterior horns

949. What is the most common treatment for a discoid meniscus?
   ➢ Partial meniscectomy and saucerization

Patella

950. Quadriceps tendon ruptures commonly occur in what age group?
   ➢ Older patients (>40 years old)
     - Remember: Above patella = Higher age

Knee

951. Patellar tendon ruptures commonly occur in what age group?
    ➢ Younger patients (<40 years old)

952. Where do patellar tendon injuries typically occur?
    ➢ Avulsion injury from the inferior pole of the patella

953. What structure may allow a patient to actively extend their knee following a ruptured patellar or quadriceps tendon?
    ➢ Intact patellar retinaculum

954. What radiographic finding may be seen with a quadriceps tendon rupture?
    ➢ Patella baja

955. What radiographic finding may be seen with a patellar tendon rupture?
    ➢ Patella alta

956. What is the Insall-Salvati ratio?
    ➢ Patellar tendon length divided by length of the patella with the knee flexed at 30°

957. Using Insall-Salvati ratio, what value suggests patella alta?
    ➢ >1.2

958. Using Insall-Salvati ratio, what value suggests patella baja?
    ➢ <0.8

959. With the knee flexed at 30°, the inferior pole of the patella should project with what radiographic line on a lateral x-ray?
    ➢ Blumensaat's line

Knee

960. The patella most commonly dislocates in which direction?
    ➤ Laterally
961. What is a "J-sign" on physical exam?
    ➤ Patella is subluxed in full extension and shifts into the trochlear groove as the knee flexes
962. What is the primary restraint to lateral patellar subluxation from 0-20° of flexion?
    ➤ Medial patellofemoral ligament (MPFL)
963. Avulsion of the MPFL most commonly occur from which location in adults?
    ➤ Femoral origin
964. What is Schottle's point?
    ➤ Femoral origin of the MPFL
965. What is the location of Schottle's point on a lateral x-ray?
    ➤ Anterior to a line drawn down the posterior femoral cortex and just proximal to the most posterior aspect of Blumensaat's line
966. What bruising pattern will you see on MRI following patellar dislocation?
    ➤ Bruising of the lateral femoral condyle and inferomedial patella
967. What is the tibial tuberosity-trochlear groove (TT-TG) measurement?
    ➤ Distance between the center of the tibial tubercle and the center of the trochlear groove
968. What is a normal TT-TG?
    ➤ <15mm

969. What procedure is performed with a large TT-TG in a patient with recurrent patellar instability?
> Tibial tubercle transfer (Fulkerson Osteotomy)

Knee

Adult Reconstruction

Total Knee Arthroplasty (TKA)

970. What is the mechanical axis of the lower extremity?
> A line drawn from the center of the femoral head to the center of the ankle joint

971. Where should the mechanical axis cross the knee in a normal patient?
> Center of the knee joint

972. What deformity is present if the mechanical axis is medial?
> Varus knee

973. What deformity is present if the mechanical axis is lateral?
> Valgus knee

974. What is the anatomic axis?
> A line drawn down the long axis of the femoral or tibial shaft

975. What is the relationship of the normal femoral anatomic axis to its mechanical axis?
> The anatomic axis is 5° lateral (more valgus) from the mechanical axis

976. What is the relationship of the normal tibial anatomic axis to its mechanical axis?
> Equal - in line with one another

977. On average, what is the slope of the proximal tibia?
> 9° of posterior slope

978. What is the Q-angle?

Knee

> An angle formed between a line connecting the ASIS to the middle of the patella and a second line connecting the tibial tubercle to the middle of the patella

979. What does the Q-angle represent?

> Directional pull of the quadriceps muscle on the patella

980. What is the difference between an apparent and an actual leg length discrepancy?

> Apparent is measured from the umbilicus to the medial malleolus

> Actual is measured from the ASIS to the medial malleolus

981. How do you perform a Rosenberg view?

> Standing PA radiograph with 45° of knee flexion

982. What are the two most common unconstrained TKA designs?

> Posterior-cruciate Retaining (CR)

> Posterior-cruciate Stabilizing (PS)

983. How can you differentiate the polyethylene insert of a PS knee and a CR knee?

> PS polyethylene will have a tibial post that engages the cam on the femoral component

984. How can you tell the difference between a PS and CR knee on lateral radiographs?

> PS knees have a box that contains the cam design
  - This makes the appearance of a filled in half moon on x-ray

> CR knees have no box and are narrower distally

Knee

- You can often see the pegs that help secure the prosthesis on lateral x-rays

985. Which type of TKA design is suitable for accepting a retrograde intramedullary nail?
   - CR knees

986. What are the indications to use a more constrained TKA?
   - Collateral ligament instability, bone loss, and sagittal plane instability

987. Which compartment is more severely diseased in a varus knee?
   - Medial compartment

988. Which compartment is more severely diseased in a valgus knee?
   - Lateral compartment

989. In a valgus knee, where does most of the wear occur?
   - Lateral distal femoral condyle
     - Results in a hypoplastic lateral femoral condyle

990. In a varus knee, where does most of the wear occur?
   - Proximal medial tibia

991. What is the most common approach for a TKA?
   - Medial parapatellar

992. What alternative approaches may be utilized for a TKA?
   - Subvastus, midvastus, or lateral parapatellar

993. What complication is more common with use of a constrained TKA?
   - Aseptic loosening

Knee

994. What is the most common complication following a TKA?
> ➤ Patellar maltracking

995. How may the components be positioned to decrease the risk of patellar maltracking?
> ➤ External rotation of the femoral and tibial components
> ➤ Lateralization of the femoral and tibial components
> ➤ Medialization of the patellar component
>> ▪ Note: When placing the patellar component intraoperatively the patella is everted – do not confuse medial and lateral

996. Why does positioning the components in this way improve patellar tracking?
> ➤ Reduces the Q-angle

997. What is Whiteside's line?
> ➤ A line drawn down the center of the trochlea to the top of the intercondylar notch

998. What is the transepicondylar axis?
> ➤ An axis between the medial and lateral femoral epicondyles

999. What is the relationship of the transepicondylar axis to Whiteside's line?
> ➤ The transepicondylar axis should be perpendicular to Whiteside's line

1000. Femoral component rotation can be referenced using what three lines?
> ➤ Whiteside's line, transepicondylar axis, and posterior condylar axis

Knee

1001. Tibial component rotation can be referenced using what two anatomic points?
   ➢ Tibial tubercle
   ➢ Tibial crest at the junction of the proximal and middle thirds of the tibia

1002. A drop rod placed in a tibial trial should line up with what anatomic structure on the foot?
   ➢ Second metatarsal

1003. What are the oblique cuts on the distal femur called?
   ➢ Chamfer

1004. When evaluating the pieces of bone removed from the distal femur in a varus knee, should the medial or lateral piece be thicker?
   ➢ Medial because the medial aspect of the distal femur is more distal

1005. When performing the proximal tibia cut, how much bone is typically removed from the diseased side (medial side of a varus knee)?
   ➢ 2mm

1006. When performing the proximal tibia cut, how much bone is typically removed from the healthy side (lateral side of a varus knee)?
   ➢ 10mm

1007. Cutting more bone from the distal femur increases which gap(s)?
   ➢ Extension gap

1008. Cutting more bone from the posterior femur increases which gap(s)?
   ➢ Flexion gap

Knee

1009. Cutting more bone from the proximal tibial increases which gap(s)?

> Flexion and extension gaps

1010. What is the order of medial releases for a varus knee?

> Deep MCL → osteophytes → Posterior Oblique Ligament → "shift and resect" osteotomy → PCL → Semimembranosus → Superficial MCL

1011. When performing lateral releases, what structures are released if there is tightness in extension?

> IT band and posterior capsule

1012. When performing lateral releases, which structure is released if there is tightness in flexion?

> Popliteus

1013. Hypersensitivity to cobalt-chrome alloy implants is likely secondary to which metal?

> Nickel

1014. What are the two common distal femur periprosthetic fracture classifications?

> Lewis and Rorabeck Classification
> - Type I: Nondisplaced fracture with well-fixed components
> - Type II: Displaced fracture with well-fixed components
> - Type III: Displaced fracture with loose components
>
> Su Classification
> - Type I: Fracture proximal to the femoral component

Knee

- Type II: Fracture originates at the anterior flange and extends proximally
- Type III: Fracture extends distal to the superior aspect of the anterior flange

1015. What is the tibial periprosthetic fracture classification?
  - Felix Classification
    - Type I: Fracture of the tibial plateau
    - Type II: Fracture around the stem
    - Type III: Fracture distal to the stem
    - Type IV: Fracture of the tibial tubercle

Unicompartmental Knee Arthroplasty (UKA)

1016. What are the indications for UKA?
  - Arthritis affecting a single compartment

1017. UKA are most commonly performed for arthritis of which compartment?
  - Medial

1018. What are the contraindications for UKA?
  - Tricompartmental arthritis, ACL deficiency, Rheumatoid arthritis, varus deformity >10°, valgus deformity >5°, flexion contracture, and recurvatum

1019. Stress fractures are most commonly seen where?
  - Around the tibial component

1020. What is the most common cause of UKA failure?
  - Degeneration of the remaining compartments

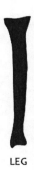
LEG

Leg

General Anatomy

1021. What nerve is at risk with proximal fibula fractures?
    > Common peroneal nerve
1022. What is Gerdy's tubercle?
    > Insertion site of the iliotibial band
1023. What shape is the mid-shaft of the tibia?
    > Triangle
1024. Where is the isthmus of the tibia?
    > Junction of the middle and distal thirds
1025. What structures are within the anterior compartment of the leg?
    > Tibialis anterior, Extensor digitormum longus (EDL), Extensor hallicus longus (EHL), Peroneus tertius, Anterior tibial artery and vein, Deep peroneal nerve
1026. What structures are within the lateral compartment of the leg?
    > Peroneus longus and brevis, Superficial peroneal nerve
1027. What structures are within the superficial posterior compartment of the leg?
    > Soleus, Gastrocnemius, and Plantaris tendon
1028. What structures are within the deep posterior compartment of the leg?
    > Flexor digitorum longus (FDL), Tibialis posterior, Flexor hallicus longus (FHL), Posterior tibial artery and vein, Tibial nerve, Peroneal artery and vein

Leg

1029. What is the first branch of the popliteal artery?
   ➢ Anterior tibial artery

1030. What is the terminal branch of the anterior tibial artery?
   ➢ Dorsalis pedis artery

1031. What is the terminal branch of the peroneal artery?
   ➢ Calcaneal branches

1032. What are the terminal branches of the posterior tibial artery?
   ➢ Medial and Lateral plantar arteries

Leg

Trauma

Tibial Shaft

1033. What are the tolerances for nonoperative management of tibial shaft fractures?
   - <10° of AP angulation
   - <5° of varus/valgus angulation
   - <1 cm of shortening
   - <10° of rotational deformity
   - >50% cortical apposition

1034. What deformity is commonly seen with proximal third tibial shaft fractures?
   - Proximal fragment:
     - Extension – Patellar tendon
     - Varus – Pes Anserine
   - Distal fragment:
     - Flexion – Gastrocnemius

1035. What is the starting point for a tibial intramedullary nail (IMN) on the AP view?
   - Medial border of the lateral tibial spine

1036. What is the starting point for a tibial IMN on the lateral view?
   - Just anterior to the articular margin

1037. What is the most common malunion deformity following use of an IMN for a proximal tibial fracture?
   - Valgus and procurvatum

1038. Where should blocking screws be placed to prevent valgus deformity?
   - Lateral to the path of the nail

1039. Where should blocking screws be placed to prevent procurvatum deformity?
- Posteriorly to the path of the nail
  - Always place the blocking screw in the concavity of the deformity you are trying to prevent

1040. What does the lateral x-ray finding of a "dreaded black line" on the anterior aspect of the tibia suggest?
- Stress fracture

1041. Spiral distal one-third tibial shaft fractures require what additional imaging?
- CT and x-rays of the ankle

1042. Why are CT and x-rays of the ankle obtained with spiral distal one-third tibial shaft fractures?
- To evaluate for posterior malleolus fractures

1043. What is the incidence of a posterior malleolus fracture with a spiral distal one-third tibial shaft fracture?
- 39%

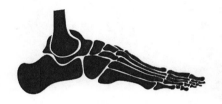

FOOT & ANKLE

Foot & Ankle

General Anatomy

1044. What nerve is at risk with ORIF of the fibula?
   ➢ Superficial peroneal nerve
1045. Where does the superficial peroneal nerve cross the fibula?
   ➢ 3-12cm proximal to the distal fibula
1046. In which direction does the superficial peroneal nerve cross the fibula?
   ➢ Posterior to anterior
1047. What nerve is at risk with open Achilles tendon repair?
   ➢ Sural
1048. Where does the sural nerve cross the Achilles tendon?
   ➢ 10cm proximal to its insertion on the calcaneus
1049. What tendon is directly medial to the Achilles tendon?
   ➢ Plantaris tendon
      - Note: do not get tricked into thinking this is a nerve intraoperatively – often referred to as the "freshman nerve"
1050. What happens to the mortise as the ankle goes from plantarflexion to dorsiflexion?
   ➢ Mortise widens
1051. What ligaments make up the syndesmosis?
   ➢ Anterior inferior tibiofibular ligament (AITFL)
   ➢ Posterior inferior tibiofibular ligament (PITFL)
   ➢ Interosseous ligament (IOL)
   ➢ Transverse tibiofibular ligament (TTFL)

Foot & Ankle

> Inferior transverse ligament (ITL)

1052. In which direction is the syndesmosis most unstable?
> Anterior to posterior

1053. The spring ligament connects which two bones?
> Calcaneus and navicular

1054. What are the primary ligaments of the medial ankle?
> Deltoid ligament, Calcaneonavicular (Spring) ligament

1055. What are the layers of the deltoid ligament?
> Superficial deltoid – attaches to the anterior colliculus of the tibia and spans the tibiotalar and subtalar joints
> Deep deltoid – originates from the posterior colliculus of the tibia and only spans the tibiotalar joint

1056. What are the primary ligaments of the lateral ankle?
> Ligaments of the syndesmosis, Anterior talofibular ligament (ATFL), Posterior talofibular ligament (PTFL), Calcaneal fibular ligament (CFL), Lateral talocalcaneal ligament (LTCL)

1057. Which lateral ankle ligament is the weakest and most likely to be injured?
> **ATF**L
  - Remember: **A**lways **T**ears **F**irst

1058. Which lateral ankle ligament is the strongest?
> PTFL

Foot & Ankle

1059. Which lateral ankle ligament is the primary restraint to inversion while the foot is in plantarflexion?
   ➢ ATFL

1060. Which lateral ankle ligament is the primary restraint to inversion while the foot is in a neutral or dorsiflexed position?
   ➢ CFL

1061. Where does the posterior tibialis tendon insert?
   ➢ Navicular and Medial cuneiform

1062. What is the function of the posterior tibialis tendon?
   ➢ Inversion and plantarflexion of the foot

1063. What is the major antagonist to the posterior tibialis tendon?
   ➢ Peroneus brevis

1064. Where does the tibialis anterior tendon insert?
   ➢ Medial cuneiform and 1st metatarsal

1065. What is the function of the tibialis anterior tendon?
   ➢ Dorsiflexion and inversion

1066. Where does the peroneus longus insert?
   ➢ 1st Metatarsal and Medial Cuneiform

1067. What is the function of the peroneus longus tendon?
   ➢ Plantarflexion and eversion

1068. Where does the peroneus brevis insert?
   ➢ 5th Metatarsal base

1069. What is the function of the peroneus brevis tendon?
   ➢ Plantarflexion and eversion

Foot & Ankle

1070. How are the peroneal tendons oriented at the level of the ankle joint?
- Peroneus brevis is anterior and Peroneus longus is posterior
    - Remember: **B**revis is closer to **B**one (fibula)

1071. What is the name of the recesses on the distal tibia where the fibula sits?
- Incisura fibularis

1072. How many muscles or tendons attach to the talus?
- Zero

1073. What percentage of the talus is covered with cartilage?
- 70%

1074. What is the blood supply of the talus?
- Artery of the tarsal canal (from the posterior tibial artery)
- Anterior tibial artery
- Artery of the tarsal sinus (from the anterior tibial and peroneal arteries)

1075. What is the main blood supply to the talus?
- Posterior tibial artery

1076. Which branch of the artery of the tarsal canal supplies the medial talar body?
- Deltoid artery

1077. What structure runs between the medial and lateral tubercles of the posterior process of the talus?
- FHL

1078. What is the primary motion of the subtalar joint?
- Inversion and eversion

Foot & Ankle

1079. What are the three facets of the subtalar joint?
   - Anterior, middle, and posterior
1080. Which facet of the calcaneus is the largest?
   - Posterior
1081. With the extensile lateral approach to the calcaneus, which structures are at risk?
   - Sural nerve
   - Lateral calcaneal branch of the peroneal artery
1082. What are the two most common approaches to the calcaneus?
   - Extensile lateral and sinus tarsi
1083. What inserts onto the base of the 5th metatarsal?
   - Peroneus brevis
   - Lateral band of the plantar fascia
1084. What is the origin of the plantar fascia?
   - Medial calcaneal tuberosity
1085. Which joints are referred to as the Chopart's joints?
   - Calcaneocuboid and talonavicular joints
1086. The Lisfranc ligament connects which two bones?
   - Medial cuneiform and the second metatarsal
1087. Which bones make up each column of the foot?
   - Medial – 1st Metatarsal, medial cuneiform, and navicular
   - Middle – 2nd and 3rd Metatarsals, middle and lateral cuneiforms
   - Lateral – 4th and 5th Metatarsals and cuboid
1088. Which column of the foot is most rigid?
   - Middle column

Foot & Ankle

1089. Which column of the foot is most flexible?
   - Lateral column

1090. Which column of the foot should not be fused?
   - Lateral column

1091. Why should the lateral column of the foot not be fused?
   - Allows for functional motion

1092. Which column of the foot carries the most load with weight bearing?
   - Medial column

1093. What muscles should be tested during a neurologic exam of the foot?
   - Tibialis anterior – ankle dorsiflexion - L4
   - Extensor hallucis longus (EHL) – great toe extension - L5
   - Gastrocnemius/Soleus complex – ankle plantarflexion - S1

1094. What are the five sensory nerves to the foot?
   - Saphenous – Medial foot
   - Deep peroneal – 1st web space
   - Superficial peroneal – Dorsum of the foot
   - Sural – Lateral foot
   - Tibial – Sole of the foot

1095. Which three vessels supply the foot?
   - Posterior tibial, Anterior tibial, and Peroneal arteries

1096. How many compartments are in the foot?
   - 9 (Medial, Lateral, 4 Interosseous, 3 Central)

1097. The sesamoids of the hallux are contained within which tendon?

> Flexor hallucis brevis (FHB)

1098. What is the purpose of the hallux sesamoids?
> Increases mechanical advantage of the FHB

1099. Which hallux sesamoid is larger?
> Tibial (medial)

1100. Which hallux sesamoid is most commonly injured?
> Tibial (medial)

1101. Which hallux sesamoid is most commonly bipartite?
> Tibial (medial)

1102. Which structure glides between the hallux sesamoids?
> Flexor hallucis longus (FHL)

1103. What structure is at risk with the medial plantar approach to the tibial sesamoid?
> Medial plantar nerve

1104. What deformity is created if both sesamoids are removed?
> Cock up deformity of the great toe

1105. What ligament is present between the 2nd through 5th metatarsals, but not between the 1st and 2nd metatarsals?
> Intermetatarsal ligament

1106. What is the name for the anatomic structure where the FDL and FHL tendons cross?
> Knot of Henry

Foot & Ankle

Trauma

Pilon

1107. What is the classification for pilon fractures?
> Ruedi and Allgower Classification
> - Type I: Non-displaced
> - Type II: Displaced fracture with no comminution
> - Type III: Comminution of the articular surface

1108. What are the 3 fragments typically encountered with a pilon fracture?
> Medial malleolus, posterolateral fragment, and anterolateral fragment

1109. What is the eponym for the posterolateral fragment?
> Volkmann fragment

1110. What attaches to the posterolateral fragment?
> Posterior inferior tibiofibular ligament (PITFL)

1111. What is the eponym for the anterolateral fragment?
> Chaput fragment

1112. Which ligament attaches to the anterolateral fragment?
> Anterior inferior tibiofibular ligament (AITFL)

1113. What is the eponym for fragment created by an AITFL avulsion off the fibula?
> Wagstaffe fragment

1114. How are high energy pilon fractures treated acutely?

Foot & Ankle

> - Splinted in the trauma bay and then stabilized with an ankle spanning external fixator
>   - Remember: Soft tissues are amenable to surgery when the skin wrinkles on exam

1115. With high energy pilon fractures, when should a CT be obtained?
> - After external fixation to allow for definitive surgical planning

1116. In which direction should the calcaneal pin be placed for an ankle spanning external fixator?
> - Medial to lateral

Ankle

1117. What is the classification for distal fibula fractures?
> - Danis-Weber Classification
>   - Weber A: Infrasyndesmotic
>   - Weber B: Transsyndesmotic
>   - Weber C: Suprasyndesmotic

1118. What is a Maisonneuve fracture?
> - Proximal third fibula fracture with associated syndesmotic injury

1119. Which type of fibula fractures have the highest association with syndesmotic injuries?
> - Weber C

1120. What provocative physical exam maneuver is indicative of syndesmotic instability?
> - Hopkin's squeeze Test

1121. Which addition x-ray should be obtained with an isolated Weber B or C fracture?

Foot & Ankle

➢ Rotational stress view

1122. What are the three ways that you can perform a stress view of the ankle?

➢ Manual external rotation stress
➢ Gravity stress
➢ Weightbearing stress

1123. How do you perform a manual external rotation stress view?

➢ Obtain a mortise x-ray of the ankle, then apply an external rotation force to the foot

1124. What does the preoperative external rotation stress test evaluate?

➢ Deltoid ligament integrity

1125. What does the intraoperative external rotation stress test evaluate following fibular fixation?

➢ Syndesmosis integrity

1126. What additional intraoperative stress maneuver can be performed to assess syndesmotic integrity?

➢ Cotton test

1127. How is the Cotton test performed?

➢ Fluoroscopic exam while pulling the fibula laterally

1128. What x-ray findings suggest syndesmotic injury?

➢ Decreased tibiofibular overlap, increased tibiofibular clear space, increased medial clear space >5mm with stress
  - Note: Increased medial clear space is due to deltoid ligament incompetence, but suggestive of syndesmotic injury

1129. What is a bimalleolar-equivalent ankle fracture?

Foot & Ankle

> Fibula fracture with widening of the medial clear space indicating an unstable ankle

1130. What is a Bosworth fracture-dislocation?

> Distal fibula fracture with a fixed posterior fibular dislocation

1131. What radiographic sign suggests restoration of fibular length?

> Dime sign

1132. What is the classification for ankle fractures?

> Lauge-Hansen Classification
>   - Supination-External Rotation (SER)
>   - SER I: AITFL sprain
>   - SER II: SER I + Weber B fibula fracture (Anteroinferior to Posterosuperior)
>   - SER III: SER II + PITFL avulsion or Posterior malleolus fracture
>   - SER IV: SER III + Deltoid ligament injury or Medial malleolus fracture
>   - Supination-Adduction (SAD)
>   - SAD I: AITFL injury or Weber A fibula fracture
>   - SAD II: SAD I + Vertical medial malleolus fracture (anteromedial impaction)
>   - Pronation-External Rotation (PER)
>   - PER I: Deltoid ligament injury or Medial malleolus fracture
>   - PER II: PER I + AITFL injury
>   - PER III: PER II + Fibula fracture (Anterosuperior to Posteroinferior)

- PER IV: PER III + PITFL avulsion or Posterior malleolus fracture
- Pronation-Abduction (PAB)
  - PAB I: Deltoid ligament injury or Medial malleolus fracture
  - PAB II: PAB I + AITFL sprain
  - PAB III: PAB II + Comminuted Weber C fibula fracture

1133. What additional imaging should be obtained with supination adduction (SAD) type injuries?
   ➤ CT of the ankle to evaluate for anteromedial impaction

1134. What are the operative indications for ankle fractures?
   ➤ Bimalleolar or bimalleolar-equivalent fractures
   ➤ Trimalleolar fractures
   ➤ >25% articular involvement of posterior malleolus fracture
   ➤ Displacement of the talus
   ➤ Displacement of an isolated medial or lateral malleolus fracture
   ➤ Bosworth fracture-dislocation
   ➤ Open fractures

1135. Fixation of a posterior malleolus fragment restores what percentage of syndesmotic stability?
   ➤ 70%

1136. What is the "Rule of 3's" for syndesmotic fixation?
   ➤ Fixate 3cm proximal to the plafond
   ➤ Capture at least 3 cortices

Foot & Ankle

- Aim 30° anterior
- Typically, a 3.5mm screw (or tightrope)

1137. How does the presence of diabetes influence the period of immobilization?

- Period of immobilization should be doubled

1138. What complication may occur if hardware is placed too distally on the posterior aspect of the fibula?

- Peroneal tendon irritation

Talus

1139. What is the classification for talar neck fractures?

- Hawkins Classification
  - Hawkins I: Non-displaced talar neck fracture
  - Hawkins II: Talar neck fracture + Subtalar dislocation
  - Hawkins III: Hawkins II + Tibiotalar dislocation
  - Hawkins IV: Hawkins III + Talonavicular dislocation

1140. What is the most common complication following a talus fracture?

- Subtalar arthritis

1141. What risk escalates with increasing severity of the Hawkins classification?

- AVN (~100% with Hawkins IV)

1142. What is Hawkins sign?

- Lucency seen along the subchondral surface of the talus on the mortise view

1143. What is the significance of the Hawkins sign?

- Revascularization of the talus

1144. When performing an ankle arthrodesis, what is the ideal position of the foot?
> Neutral dorsiflexion, 5-10° of external rotation (helps clear foot when ambulating), and 5° hindfoot valgus

1145. What talus fracture is commonly seen in snowboarders?
> Lateral process fracture

Subtalar Dislocations

1146. Are medial or lateral subtalar dislocations more common?
> Medial

1147. Which structures may block the reduction of a medial subtalar dislocation?
> Lateral structures – Peroneal tendons, EDB, and Talonavicular joint capsule

1148. Which structures may block the reduction of a lateral subtalar dislocation?
> Medial structures – Posterior tibialis tendon, FHL, and FDL
> - Most commonly Posterior tibialis tendon

1149. What associated fracture most commonly occurs with lateral subtalar dislocations?
> Cuboid fracture

1150. What other joint commonly dislocates with subtalar joint dislocations?
> Talonavicular joint

Foot & Ankle

Calcaneus

1151. What are the classifications for calcaneus fractures?
> ➢ Sanders Classification
>> ▪ Type I: Non-displaced posterior facet
>> ▪ Type II: One fracture line (2 fragments)
>> ▪ Type III: Two fracture lines (3 fragments)
>> ▪ Type IV: Comminuted (≥4 fragments)
> ➢ Essex-Lopresti Classification
>> ▪ Tongue type
>> ▪ Joint depression type

1152. On what imaging is the Sanders Classification based?
> ➢ Coronal CT at the widest portion of the posterior facet

1153. What deformity is commonly seen with a calcaneus fracture?
> ➢ Shortening, widening, and varus

1154. What is an urgent concern with a displaced tongue type calcaneus fracture?
> ➢ Posterior skin necrosis

1155. In what position should a tongue type fracture be splinted?
> ➢ Plantarflexion

1156. What are the two primary fragments for intra-articular calcaneus fractures?
> ➢ Superomedial (constant) fragment
> ➢ Superolateral fragment

1157. Why is the superomedial fragment referred to as the constant fragment?

> Does not typically displace due to the deltoid and talocalcaneal ligaments

1158. What is Bohler's angle?
    > An angle created by lines drawn from the top of the posterior tuberosity and anterior processes to the top of the posterior facet

1159. What is a normal Bohler's angle?
    > 20-40°

1160. What is the Critical Angle of Gissane?
    > An angle created by the intersection of the posterior facet and the anterior process

1161. What is a normal Critical Angle of Gissane?
    > 130-145°

1162. How will collapse of the posterior facet influence Bohler's angle?
    > Decreases Bohler's angle

1163. How will collapse of the posterior facet influence the Critical Angle of Gissane?
    > Increases the Critical Angle of Gissane

1164. What are the operative indications for calcaneus fractures?
    > Displaced tongue-type, Sanders II-IV, anterior process fracture disrupting the CC joint, joint depression, sustentaculum tali displacement

1165. What is the recommended treatment for a Sanders IV calcaneus fracture?
    > Primary subtalar arthrodesis

Foot & Ankle

1166. What structure is at risk with a screw that is placed from lateral to medial at the level of the sustentaculum tali?
> FHL

Lisfranc

1167. The foot is commonly in what position when a Lisfranc injury occurs?
> Axial compression of a plantarflexed foot

1168. Which part of the Lisfranc ligament is the strongest?
> Interosseous

1169. What radiographic sign is indicative of a Lisfranc injury?
> Fleck sign – avulsion of the Lisfranc ligament from the 2nd metatarsal

1170. What makes the Lisfranc joint inherently stable?
> Recessed 2nd metatarsal due to the more proximal middle cuneiform – "Keystone"

1171. What physical exam finding heightens your suspicion of a Lisfranc injury?
> Plantar ecchymosis

1172. What radiograph should be obtained with a suspected Lisfranc injury?
> Weight-bearing x-rays of both feet

1173. Displacement typically occurs in which direction?
> Dorsal due to the weaker dorsal ligaments

1174. How are Lisfranc injuries treated surgically?
> ORIF or arthrodesis

1175. Which treatment is recommended for a purely ligamentous Lisfranc injury?
   ➢ Arthrodesis
1176. How does ORIF differ from arthrodesis?
   ➢ ORIF – the joint surfaces are maintained
   ➢ Arthrodesis – cartilage is removed from the joint surface to allow for fusion
1177. In general, what is the direction of fixation for Lisfranc injuries?
   ➢ Proximal to distal and medial to lateral

5th Metatarsal

1178. What are the zones of the 5th metatarsal?
   ➢ Zone 1: Proximal tubercle
   ➢ Zone 2: Metaphyseal/diaphyseal junction
   ➢ Zone 3: Diaphysis, distal to the intermetatarsal articulation
1179. What is the eponym for a Zone 1 fracture?
   ➢ Pseudo-Jones
1180. What is the eponym for a Zone 2 fracture?
   ➢ Jones fracture
1181. Fractures in which zone have an increased risk for nonunion?
   ➢ Zone 2 – vascular watershed area
1182. Which 5th metatarsal base fractures are typically treated surgically?
   ➢ Zone 2 or 3 fractures in athletes
1183. What is the starting point for an intramedullary screw to treat a 5th metatarsal fracture?
   ➢ "High and inside"

Foot & Ankle

Foot & Ankle Conditions

Achilles Tendon

1184. What physical exam test should be performed to assess the integrity of the Achilles tendon?
> Thompson test

1185. How do you perform the Thompson test?
> Patient prone, squeeze the calf and evaluate for ankle plantarflexion

1186. What class of antibiotics have been associated with Achilles tendon ruptures?
> Fluoroquinolones

1187. Where does the Achilles tendon typically rupture?
> 6cm proximal to its insertion – vascular watershed area

1188. What is the difference between ankle plantarflexion strength following nonoperative and operative treatment of Achilles tendon ruptures?
> None, equivalent plantarflexion strength

1189. Which tendon can be transferred to augment an Achilles tendon repair in the setting of a chronic rupture?
> FHL

1190. What is the Silfverskiöld test?
> A test to evaluate the gastrocnemius-soleus complex and ankle equinus

1191. How is the Silfverskiöld test performed?
> Evaluate ankle dorsiflexion while immobilizing the subtalar and talonavicular joints with the hip

and knee extended and again with the hip and knee flexed

1192. What does the Silfverskiöld test indicate?
> Differentiates whether the equinus contracture is due to isolated contracture of the gastrocnemius tendon or from the gastrocnemius-soleus complex (heel cord)

1193. What would you find while performing the Silfverskiöld test in a patient with an isolated gastrocnemius contracture?
> Increased ankle dorsiflexion with hip and knee flexion
  - Gastrocnemius crosses both the knee and ankle joints. Flexing the knee takes away the pull from the gastrocnemius allowing increased ankle dorsiflexion

Peroneal Tendons

1194. What is the primary restraint to peroneal tendon dislocation?
> Superior peroneal retinaculum

1195. Which tendon most commonly develops tears from recurrent peroneal tendon subluxation?
> Peroneus brevis

1196. What provocative maneuver can be performed in a patient with suspected peroneal tendon dislocation?
> Apprehension test: Dorsiflexion and eversion against resistance causes the sensation of tendon subluxation

Foot & Ankle

1197. What condition presents similar to a peroneal tendon dislocation, but demonstrates no tendon instability on physical exam?
   ➢ Peroneus brevis tear

Posterior Tibial Tendon Insufficiency (PTTI)

1198. What are the stages of PTTI?
   ➢ Stage I: Normal
   ➢ Stage II: Flatfoot, unable to perform single-heel rise
   ➢ Stage III: Stage II + "too many toes" sign
   ➢ Stage IV: Stage III + Deltoid ligament involvement + Talar tilt

1199. What is the most common cause of adult flatfoot deformity?
   ➢ PTTI

1200. Which ligament is attenuated with PTTI?
   ➢ Superomedial calcaneonavicular (Spring) ligament

1201. How does the posterior tibial tendon affect the transverse tarsal joints?
   ➢ Locks the transverse tarsal joint creating a rigid joint for toe-off

1202. What is the "too many toes" sign?
   ➢ Visibility of the lesser toes when viewing the heel from behind

1203. What does the "too many toes" sign indicate?
   ➢ Forefoot abduction

1204. What brace is typically used in nonoperative management of PTTI?
> Ankle-Foot-Orthosis (AFO)

Hallux Valgus

1205. What is the eponym for hallux valgus?
> Bunion

1206. What is the deforming force that pulls the great toe into valgus?
> Adductor hallucis

1207. What happens to the sesamoid complex?
> Translates laterally

1208. What other condition may result secondary to lateral translation of the sesamoid complex?
> Transfer metatarsalgia: Overloading of the lesser metatarsal heads

1209. Displacement of the abductor hallucis leads to what deformity of the great toe?
> Plantarflexion and pronation

1210. What is the Hallux Valgus Angle (HVA)?
> Angle created between the first metatarsal and proximal phalanx
  - Normal: ≤15°

1211. What is the Intermetatarsal Angle (IMA)?
> Angle created by the shafts of the first and second metatarsals
  - Normal: ≤ 9°

1212. What is the Distal Metatarsal Articulation Angle (DMAA)?

Foot & Ankle

> - Angle between a line drawn perpendicular to the long axis of the first metatarsal and the articular cap of the first metatarsal head
>   - Normal: ≤10°

1213. What are the indications for a distal metatarsal osteotomy?

> - HVA ≤40°, IMA ≤13°

1214. What are the indications for a proximal or combined osteotomy?

> - HVA >40°, IMA >13°

1215. What treatment is indicated with first tarsometatarsal joint (TMTJ) arthritis or instability?

> - First TMTJ arthrodesis

1216. What complication may occur from overcorrection?

> - Hallux varus

1217. What deformity may occur with injury to the FHL?

> - Cock-up deformity

Hallux Rigidus

1218. What is hallux rigidus?

> - Degenerative arthritis of the first metatarsophalangeal joint (MTPJ) resulting in loss of motion

1219. What movements exacerbate pain in hallux rigidus?

> - Push-off and forced great toe dorsiflexion

1220. Where do osteophytes typically develop?

> - Dorsally

1221. How does pain with motion correlate with disease severity?
> ➤ Pain with extremes of motion indicates milder disease
> ➤ Pain with mid-range motion indicates more severe disease

1222. Pain with terminal dorsiflexion may benefit from what procedure?
> ➤ Dorsal cheilectomy
>   - Note: Contraindicated in patient with pain in mid-range of motion

1223. What is the most commonly performed procedure for hallux rigidus?
> ➤ Arthrodesis

Cavovarus Foot

1224. What deformities characterize a cavovarus foot?
> ➤ Cavus
> ➤ Hindfoot varus
> ➤ Plantarflexion of the first ray
> ➤ Forefoot pronation and adduction

1225. What is the most common cause of a cavovarus foot?
> ➤ Neurologic conditions

1226. What neurologic condition is the most common cause of bilateral cavovarus deformities?
> ➤ Charcot-Marie-Tooth (CMT)

1227. What must be ruled-out in the presence of new onset unilateral cavovarus?
> ➤ Spinal cord tumor or tethering

Foot & Ankle

1228. Which muscles are weak in a cavovarus foot?
> Tibialis anterior and Peroneus brevis

1229. The weak tibialis anterior is overpowered by which muscle?
> Peroneus longus

1230. The weak peroneus brevis is overpowered by which muscle?
> Posterior tibialis

1231. Stress fractures to which bone can be seen with a cavovarus deformity?
> 5th metatarsal

1232. Contracture of which muscle is commonly seen in the setting of a cavovarus foot?
> Gastrocnemius

1233. What procedure may be indicated to address concomitant ankle equinus?
> Gastrocnemius recession or tendoachilles lengthening (TAL)

1234. Elevation of the medial arch leads to contracture of which structure?
> Plantar fascia

1235. What is the talocalcaneal angle?
> Angle between the long axis of the talus and the calcaneus on the AP view of the foot

1236. What is a normal talocalcaneal angle?
> 20-40°

1237. What talocalcaneal angle suggests hindfoot varus?
> <20°

1238. What is the Coleman block test?
> A block placed under the lateral aspect of the foot assesses the flexibility of hindfoot varus

1239. A varus hindfoot that corrects to neutral with Coleman block testing is caused by what part of the foot?
> Forefoot driven

1240. What soft-tissue procedure is performed to correct first ray plantarflexion?
> Peroneus longus to brevis transfer

1241. What tendon transfer can be performed to address the weak Tibialis anterior?
> Posterior tibial tendon transfer to the dorsum of the foot

Freiberg's Disease

1242. What is Freiberg's disease?
> Avascular necrosis of the metatarsal head

1243. Freiberg's disease occurs most commonly in which metatarsal?
> Second

1244. Which metatarsals are the least commonly involved?
> Fourth and fifth

1245. What is thought to be a risk factor for Freiberg's disease?
> Long second metatarsal

Foot & Ankle

Lesser Toes

1246. What deformities are seen with claw toes?
   ➤ MTPJ hyperextension with PIPJ and DIPJ flexion

1247. What toe deformity is commonly seen following missed compartment syndrome of the foot?
   ➤ Claw toes

1248. What deformities are seen with hammertoes?
   ➤ Neutral MTPJ with PIPJ flexion and DIPJ extension

1249. Over-pull of which tendon leads to hammer toe deformity?
   ➤ EDL

1250. What deformity is seen with mallet toes?
   ➤ Hyperflexion of the DIPJ

1251. Contracture of which tendon leads to a mallet toe deformity?
   ➤ FDL

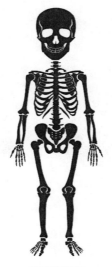

PEDIATRICS

Pediatrics

General Anatomy

1252. What are the zones of the physis?
- Resting/Reserve
- Proliferative
- Hypertrophic
  - Maturation, Degeneration, and Zone of provisional calcification
- Metaphysis
  - Primary Spongiosa, Secondary spongiosa

1253. Through which zone of the physis do Salter Harris fractures occur?
- Hypertrophic zone (Zone of provisional calcification)

1254. What is the Groove of Ranvier?
- Germinal cells that are continuous with the physis and contribute to circumferential growth

1255. What structure anchors the periphery of the physis?
- Perichondrial Ring of La Croix

1256. What is the major source of nutrition for the growth plate?
- Perichondral artery

1257. What percentage of growth occurs from the proximal and distal ends of the clavicle, humerus, radius/ulna, femur and tibia/fibula?
- Clavicle
  - Proximal: 80%
  - Distal: 20%

Pediatrics

- Humerus
  - Proximal: 80%
  - Distal: 20%
- Radius/Ulna
  - Proximal: 25%
  - Distal: 75%
- Femur
  - Proximal: 25%
  - Distal: 75%
- Tibia/Fibula
  - Proximal: 55%
  - Distal: 45%

1258. How much growth occurs per year at each physis in the lower extremity? What is this as a percentage of lower extremity growth?

- Proximal femur: 3mm (10%)
- Distal femur: 9mm (40%)
- Proximal tibia: 6mm (30%)
- Distal tibia: 5mm (20%)

1259. Describe the direction of closure of the proximal tibial physis?

- Posteromedial to anterolateral
- Proximal to distal

1260. Describe the direction of closure of the distal tibial physis?

- Central to medial to lateral

1261. Which joints have intraarticular metaphyses?

- **S**houlder, **H**ip, **E**lbow, **A**nkle
  - Remember: "**SHEA**"

Pediatrics

1262. How does the blood supply to the femoral head change with age?
- Patient <4 years old: Contributions from the Medial and lateral femoral circumflex arteries, and the Artery of ligamentum teres
- Patient ≥4 years old: Primary blood supply is the Medial femoral circumflex artery

1263. What is the order of ossification of the pediatric elbow? At what age does each center ossify?
- **C**apitellum – 1 year old
- **R**adial head – 3 years old
- Medial "**I**nternal" epicondyle – 5 years old
- **T**rochlea – 7 years old
- **O**lecranon – 9 years old
- Lateral "**E**xternal" epicondyle – 11 years old
  - Remember: **"C-R-I-T-O-E"**

1264. What is the order of fusion of the pediatric elbow? At what age does each center fuse?
- **T**rochlea – 12 years old
- **L**ateral epicondyle – 12 years old
- **C**oronoid – 12 years old
- **O**lecranon – 15 years old
- **R**adial head – 15 years old
- **Me**dial epicondyle – 17 years old
  - Remember: **"TLC OR Me"**

1265. Which epiphyseal centers are present at birth?
- Distal **F**emur
- Proximal **T**ibia
- **C**alcaneus
- Proximal **H**umerus

- > Talus
- > Cuboid
  - Remember: "**F**ull **T**erm **C**hildren **H**ave **T**hese **C**enters"

1266. What muscles cause avulsion fractures of the ASIS, AIIS, Ischial tuberosity and Lesser trochanter?
- > ASIS: Sartorius
- > AIIS: Rectus femoris
- > Ischial tuberosity: Hamstring
- > Lesser trochanter: Iliopsoas

Pediatrics

The Basics

Physis

1267. What is the classification for fractures involving the physis?
> Salter Harris Classification
> - SH I: Fracture through the physis
> - SH II: Fracture through the physis with extension into the metaphysis
> - SH III: Fracture through the physis with extension into the epiphysis
> - SH IV: Fracture through the metaphysis, physis and epiphysis
> - SH V: Physeal crush injury

1268. Overall, what is the most common type of Salter Harris fracture?
> SH II

1269. What is the most common SH fracture in the distal fibula, distal radius, distal tibia, and distal femur?
> Distal Fibula: SH I
> Distal Radius: SH II
> Distal Tibia: SH III
> Distal Femur: SH IV

1270. Which type of Salter Harris fracture has the highest incidence of growth arrest?
> SH IV
> - Distal femur: 50%
> - Distal ulna: 50%

Pediatrics

1271. What is a Thurston-Holland fragment?
> ➤ Metaphyseal fragment of a SH II fracture

1272. What is the Risser Classification?
> ➤ Measure of skeletal maturity based on the ossification of the iliac apophysis. Stages start laterally and progress medially
>   - Stage 1: ≤25% of the ilium is ossified
>   - Stage 2: 50% ossified
>   - Stage 3: 75% ossified
>   - Stage 4: 100% ossified
>   - Stage 5: Fusion, apophysis to the iliac crest

1273. When performing an epiphysiodesis, should you err on being too close to the epiphysis or metaphysis?
> ➤ Epiphysis, this is closer to the proliferative zone where the germinal cells are found

1274. As a general rule, at what age do boys and girls stop growing in their lower extremities?
> ➤ Boys: 16 years old
> ➤ Girls: 14 years old

1275. What are the indications for a physeal bar excision?
> ➤ <50% physeal involvement
> ➤ ≥2 years of growth remaining

Joint Hypermobility

1276. What scoring system is used for generalized soft tissue laxity?
> ➤ Beighton Score
>   - Passive hyperextension of the small finger >90° (1 point each side)

- Passive abduction of the thumb to the volar forearm (1 point each side)
- Hyperextension of the knee >10° (1 point each side)
- Hyperextension of the elbow >10° (1 point each side)
- Palms touch the ground with forward bending at the waist while knees extended (1 point)

1277. Based on the Beighton score, what defines hypermobility?
> Score ≥5 out of 9

Lower Extremity Alignment

1278. How does the physiologic alignment of the lower extremity change with age?
> Salenius Curve
> - Birth–1.5 years old: Genu varum
> - 2 years old: Neutral alignment
> - >2 years old: Genu valgum
>   - Maximum genu valgum at 3 years of age
> - Adult alignment of slight valgus at 6-8 years of age

1279. What are the three conditions that can cause in-toeing?
> Femoral anteversion, Internal tibial torsion, and Metatarsus adductus

1280. Which cause of in-toeing is most common in infants? Toddlers? Children?
> Infants: Metatarsus adductus
> Toddlers: Internal tibial torsions

Pediatrics

> Children: Femoral anteversion

1281. A patient who "W" sits likely has what rotational abnormality of the lower extremities?
> Increased femoral anteversion

1282. The thigh-foot angle is used to evaluate which aspect of the lower extremity rotational profile?
> Tibial torsion

1283. What is miserable malalignment syndrome?
> Increased femoral anteversion and external tibial torsion

Cerebral Palsy (CP)

1284. What is CP?
> A nonprogressive upper motor neuron disease that occurs following injury to the developing brain

1285. What classification is used to grade patient mobility in CP?
> GMFCS (Gross Motor Functional Classification Scale)
> - Level I: Independent ambulator, almost normal motor function
> - Level II: Walks independently, difficulty outside of the home
> - Level III: Walks with assistance
> - Level IV: Severely limited, wheelchair bound
> - Level V: Nonambulatory, needs assistance with all aspect of life

1286. What is the difference between quadriplegic, diplegic, and hemiplegic CP?

- Quadriplegic: Total body involvement
- Diplegic: Lower extremities affected more than upper extremities
- Hemiplegic: Involves one side of the body

Upper Extremity

Little Leaguer's Shoulder

1287. What is Little Leaguer's Shoulder?
   ➤ SH I proximal humerus overuse injury

1288. What is the most common factor leading to Little Leaguer's Shoulder?
   ➤ Pitch count

1289. What radiographic finding is suggestive of Little Leaguer's Shoulder?
   ➤ Widening of the proximal humeral physis

Supracondylar Humerus

1290. What is the classification for supracondylar humerus fractures?
   ➤ Gartland Classification
     - Type I: Nondisplaced
     - Type II: Displaced, intact posterior periosteal hinge
     - Type III: Completely displaced, no intact posterior hinge

1291. Are flexion or extension type supracondylar humerus fractures more common?
   ➤ Extension (98%)

1292. What is the most common neurologic injury with extension type supracondylar humerus fractures?
   ➤ AIN palsy

Pediatrics

1293. Supracondylar humerus fractures that displace in which direction have a higher association with AIN palsies?
   ➢ Posterolateral

1294. What is the second most common neurologic injury associated with extension type fractures?
   ➢ Radial nerve palsy

1295. Supracondylar humerus fractures that displace in which direction have a higher association with radial nerve palsies?
   ➢ Posteromedial

1296. What is the most common neurologic injury seen with flexion type fractures?
   ➢ Ulnar nerve palsy

1297. If you see ecchymosis anteromedially, what direction is the supracondylar humerus fracture displaced?
   ➢ Posterolaterally. Ecchymosis, if present, is opposite the displacement. Occurs due to stretching of the skin and soft tissues

1298. What radiographic sign might you see with a subtle Type I supracondylar humerus fracture?
   ➢ Posterior fat pad sign

1299. What radiographic line should you check on the lateral radiograph when evaluating elbow injuries?
   ➢ Anterior humeral line, it should intersect the middle third of the ossified capitellum in patients ≥5 years old

1300. What is Bauman's angle?
> Measurement for coronal displacement on the AP radiograph

1301. How do you measure Bauman's angle?
> Angle between a line drawn down the anatomic axis of the humerus and a line along the lateral condylar physis
- Normal: 70-75°

1302. What is the usual treatment for a Type I supracondylar humerus fracture?
> Long arm cast

1303. How are Type II and Type III supracondylar humerus fractures typically treated?
> Closed reduction and percutaneous pinning (CRPP)

1304. What is a general rule of thumb for how many pins should be used for Type II and Type III supracondylar humerus fractures?
> Type II – 2 pins
> Type III – 3 pins

1305. Which structure is at risk when placing a medial pin?
> Ulnar nerve

1306. What deformity most commonly occurs following malunion?
> Cubitus Varus (Gunstock deformity) – mostly an aesthetic deformity

1307. Development of cubitus varus increases the risk of which fracture in the future?
> Lateral condyle fractures

Pediatrics

Elbow

1308. Is the medial epicondyle an anterior or posterior structure?
    ➢ Posterior

1309. What additional elbow injury commonly occurs in concert with medial epicondyle fractures?
    ➢ Elbow dislocation

1310. What additional x-ray views are recommended to evaluate medial epicondyle fractures?
    ➢ Internal oblique and distal humerus axial views

1311. What are the operative indications for medial epicondyle fractures?
    ➢ Displacement >5mm, entrapment within the joint, open, ulnar nerve entrapment, gross elbow instability

1312. What reduction maneuver can be attempted to reduce an incarcerated medial epicondyle fracture?
    ➢ Roberts Maneuver: Valgus stress with forearm supination and wrist extension

1313. An olecranon apophyseal fracture in small children is pathognomonic for what condition?
    ➢ Osteogenesis Imperfecta

1314. A reported "elbow dislocation" in a child <3 years old is more likely to be what other injury?
    ➢ Distal humeral physeal separation

1315. In which direction do distal humeral physeal separations most commonly occur?
    ➢ Posteromedial
        ▪ Remember: Elbow dislocation are most commonly posterolateral

Pediatrics

1316. What is the most common radial neck fracture classification in children?
> O'brien Classification
- Type I: <30° angulation
- Type 2: 30-60° angulation
- Type 3: >60° angulation

1317. What associated condition should be ruled out in the setting of radial neck fractures?
> Compartment Syndrome of the volar forearm

1318. What complications can occur following ORIF of a radial neck fracture with extensive dissection?
> Radioulnar synostosis
> Avascular necrosis (AVN) of the radial head

1319. Lateral overgrowth at the elbow is a common occurrence following what injury?
> Lateral condyle fractures

1320. What neurologic complication can occur following lateral condyle fractures?
> Tardy ulnar nerve palsy

1321. What is a nursemaid's elbow?
> Subluxation of the radial head from the annular ligament

1322. What is the reduction maneuver for a nursemaid's elbow?
> Supination and flexion or hyperpronation in a flexed position

Pediatrics

Forearm & Wrist

1323. What are the tolerances for both bone forearm fractures (BBFF)?
- ≤9 years old
  - Angulation: <15°
  - Rotation: <45°
  - Bayonet apposition: <1cm
- >9 years old
  - Proximal 1/3:
    - Angulation: <10°
    - Rotation: 0°
  - Distal 2/3:
    - Angulation: <15°
    - Rotation: <30°
  - No bayonet apposition is acceptable >9 years old

1324. What is a greenstick fracture?
- Incomplete fracture with an intact cortex

1325. What is the reduction maneuver for an apex volar fracture? Apex dorsal fracture?
- Apex volar: Pronate the forearm
- Apex dorsal: Supinate the forearm
  - Remember: Always rotate the thumb towards the apex of the deformity

1326. What is a buckle (torus) fracture?
- An incomplete compression fracture at the junction between the cortical and metaphyseal bone
- Must have two points of inflection in the cortex

Pediatrics

1327. What are some important characteristics of a good long arm cast?
> 3-point mold, interosseous mold, straight ulnar border, supracondylar mold, ulnar deviation

1328. What is a cast index?
> Sagittal width of the cast divided by the coronal width of the cast

1329. What value should the cast index be?
> <0.8, associated with a lower chance of losing reduction

Hand

1330. What is a Seymour fracture?
> Open distal phalanx fracture with germinal matrix interposition

1331. What complications commonly occur following Seymour fractures?
> Infection, nail plate deformity, physeal arrest

1332. How long after injury is a Seymour fracture considered chronic?
> >24 hours

1333. Finger syndactyly most commonly occurs between which two digits?
> Middle and ring fingers

1334. What constitutes a complex syndactyly?
> Sharing of bone or nail plate between two digits

1335. What makes a syndactyly complete or incomplete?
> Whether or not the skin bridge extends the entire length of the digit

Pediatrics

1336. What is the most common complication following syndactyly release?
> Web creep

1337. What is preaxial polydactyly?
> Thumb duplication

1338. What is the classification for preaxial polydactyly?
> Wassel Classification
- Type I: Bifid distal phalanx
- Type II: Duplicated distal phalanx
- Type III: Bifid proximal phalanx
- Type IV: Duplicated proximal phalanx
- Type V: Bifid metacarpal
- Type VI: Duplicated metacarpal
- Type VII: Triphalangeal thumb

1339. What is postaxial polydactyly?
> Extra rudimentary digit or nubbin on the ulnar aspect of the hand

1340. Postaxial polydactyly is most common in which ethnicity?
> African Americans

1341. What is camptodactyly?
> Flexion deformity of the finger

1342. What tendon is involved with pediatric trigger thumb?
> FPL

1343. What is the name of the nodule commonly palpable with pediatric trigger thumb?
> Notta's node

Upper Extremity Syndromes & Conditions

1344. What is Madelung's deformity?
   - ➤ Disruption of the volar ulnar third of the distal radial physis

1345. What condition is commonly associated with an undescended scapula?
   - ➤ Sprengel's deformity

1346. Pseudarthrosis of the clavicle is most commonly seen on which side?
   - ➤ Right side
     - Note: Found on the left side with situs inversus

1347. What is believed to contribute to pseudarthrosis of the clavicle?
   - ➤ Pulsatile compression from the subclavian artery

Pediatrics

Spine

Scoliosis

1348. How do you name a scoliotic curve?
 ➢ Named for the direction of convexity

1349. Early onset scoliosis occurs before what age?
 ➢ 10 years old

1350. At what ages do infantile, juvenile and adolescent scoliosis occur?
 ➢ Infantile: <3 years old
 ➢ Juvenile: 3-10 years old
 ➢ Adolescent: >10 years old

1351. How do you measure a Cobb angle?
 ➢ A line is drawn along the superior end plate of the most proximally tilted vertebrae. A second line is drawn on the inferior end plate of the most tilted vertebrae distally. Perpendicular lines are then drawn to these two lines and the angle of intersection is measured

1352. A scoliometer reading of 7° (rotational) is associated with what degree of coronal plane abnormality?
 ➢ 20°

1353. What is the difference between scoliosis and spinal asymmetry?
 ➢ Spinal asymmetry <10° curve
 ➢ Scoliosis ≥10° curve

1354. How do you determine the stable vertebrae and the neutral vertebrae when evaluating an x-ray?

Pediatrics

- Stable vertebrae: Most proximal vertebrae that is bisected by the central sacral vertical line (CSVL)
- Neutral vertebrae: Neutrally rotated, equal distance between pedicles

1355. Thoracic scoliosis most commonly occurs in which direction?
- Right

1356. What imaging modality should be obtained in any patient with an atypical scoliotic curve (ie. left thoracic curve)?
- MRI of the spine to evaluate for intraspinal pathology such as tethered cord, Chiari malformation, or syrinx

1357. Are larger curves more common in males or females?
- Females

1358. What is the best predictor of curve progression?
- Peak growth velocity

1359. When does peak growth velocity occur in regards to Risser staging?
- Before Risser Stage 1

1360. Describe the basic treatment based on curve severity?
- 0-24°: Observation
- 25-49°: Bracing
- ≥ 50°: Surgery

1361. What curve magnitude is associated with cardiopulmonary dysfunction?
- >90°

Pediatrics

1362. What thoracic and lumbar curve magnitudes have a high association with progression in a skeletally mature patient?
> Thoracic: >50°
> Lumbar: >30°

1363. What is the goal of bracing as a treatment modality?
> To stop curve progression in skeletally immature patients

1364. How many hours a day must the brace actually be worn to prevent progression?
> Minimum of 13 hours/day

1365. What is crankshaft phenomenon?
> Progressive rotational and angular deformity after segmental posterior spinal fusion

1366. In congenital scoliosis, what deformity progresses most rapidly?
> Unsegmented bar with hemivertebrae

Kyphosis

1367. What is normal thoracic kyphosis?
> 20-40°

1368. What is Scheuermann's Kyphosis?
> Rigid thoracic kyphosis of >45°

1369. What radiographic finding must be present to diagnose Scheuermann's?
> Anterior wedging of >5° in 3 consecutive vertebrae

1370. What additional radiographic finding is seen at the endplates in Scheuermann's Kyphosis?

Pediatrics

> Schmorl's nodes – protrusions into the vertebral body from the disk space

Spondylolysis/Spondylolisthesis

1371. What is spondylolysis?
> Anatomic defect of the pars interarticularis without vertebral body displacement

1372. What radiographic finding is seen with spondylolysis?
> Scotty dog sign

1373. On what radiograph are the pars defect and Scotty dog sign identified?
> Oblique

1374. What is spondylolisthesis?
> Forward translation of one vertebral segment relative to the next caudal segment

1375. How is spondylolisthesis classified?
> Meyerding Classification
> - Grade I: <25%
> - Grade II: 25-49%
> - Grade III: 50-75%
> - Grade IV: >75-100%
> - Grade V: Spondyloptosis

1376. What is spondyloptosis?
> Complete, >100% slippage of a vertebral body anteriorly to the next caudal segment

1377. What level does spondylolisthesis most commonly occur?
> L5/S1

Pediatrics

1378. What physical exam maneuver will elicit pain in a patient with spondylolisthesis?
> Lumbar extension

1379. What sports may predispose patients to spondylolysis?
> Sports with lumbar hyperextension – gymnastics, diving, football, and rowing

1380. What muscle group is most commonly spastic with acute spondylolisthesis?
> Hamstrings

Lower Extremity

Developmental Dysplasia of the Hip (DDH)

1381. What is DDH?
   ➢ Abnormal acetabular development resulting in a shallow socket with femoral head subluxation or dislocation
1382. What patients are at risk for developing DDH?
   ➢ First born, female, breech positioning, positive family history
1383. What other conditions should also be looked for in a patient with DDH?
   ➢ Torticollis, clubfoot, metatarsus adductus
      - "Packaging disorders"
1384. In typical DDH, where is the acetabular deficiency?
   ➢ Anterolateral
1385. What radiograph can be obtained to evaluate anterior femoral head coverage?
   ➢ False profile view
1386. In spastic DDH, where is the acetabular deficiency?
   ➢ Posterosuperior
1387. What 2 physical exam maneuvers are used to test for DDH in patients <3 months of age?
   ➢ Ortolani: Abduction and elevation of the femur (reduces dislocated hip)
   ➢ Barlow: Adduction and depression of the femur (dislocates hip)
      - Remember: **B**arlow pushes **B**ackwards

Pediatrics

1388. What is the Galeazzi sign?
> Apparent limb length discrepancy noted at the top of the knees when the patient is supine with the hips and knees flexed to 90°
> - DDH, congenital short femur, and proximal femoral deficiency may all cause a positive Galeazzi sign

1389. What is the primary imaging modality for DDH in patients <6 months of age?
> Ultrasound

1390. What is the alpha angle?
> Measurement of the bony acetabulum on ultrasound
> - Normal is >60°

1391. At what age does the femoral head begin to ossify?
> 4-6 months

1392. What is Hilgenreiner's line?
> Horizontal line through the triradiate cartilage bilaterally

1393. Where should the normal femoral head be in relation to Hilgenreiner's line?
> Femoral head should be inferior

1394. What is Perkin's line?
> Vertical line, perpendicular to Hilgenreiner's line on the most lateral aspect of the acetabulum

1395. Where should the normal femoral head be in relation to Perkin's line?
> Femoral head should be medial

Pediatrics

1396. What is Shenton's line?
    - A smooth line drawn from the inferior femoral neck and continuing along the superior aspect of the obturator foramen
1397. What is the acetabular index (AI)?
    - Angle formed by Hilgenreiner's line and the lateral edge of the acetabulum
1398. What is normal AI?
    - <25°
        - Remember: AI should be 24° by 24 months
1399. What is the Center Edge Angle (CEA)?
    - Angle formed by a vertical line centered in the femoral head and the lateral aspect of the acetabulum
1400. What is normal CEA?
    - >20°
1401. What is the initial treatment of DDH for a patient <6 months old?
    - Pavlik harness
1402. What is the success rate of treatment in a Pavlik harness?
    - 90%
1403. What complication is seen with Pavlik harnesses applied in too much abduction?
    - Femoral head AVN if >60° of abduction
1404. What complications are seen with Pavlik harnesses applied in too much flexion?
    - Transient femoral nerve palsy if flexed >100°
    - Inferior subluxation of the femoral head

Pediatrics

1405. What radiographic finding would indicate femoral head AVN following treatment in a Pavlik harness?
> No radiographic evidence of the ossific nucleus of the femoral head 1 year after initiation of treatment

1406. What are the potential obstacles to reduction of a dislocated hip?
> Iliopsoas tendon
> Labrum
> Hypertrophied ligamentum teres
> Pulvinar
> Transverse acetabular ligament
> Hourglass capsule
> Adductors
> Bony anatomy
  - Acetabular dysplasia
  - Femoral version

Legg-Calve-Perthes

1407. What is Perthes?
> Idiopathic AVN of the proximal femoral epiphysis

1408. What is the classification for Perthes?
> Herring Classification (Lateral Pillar) – based on AP radiograph
  - Group A: Full height of the lateral pillar of the epiphysis
  - Group B: >50% height maintained
  - Group C: <50% height maintained

Pediatrics

1409. Is Perthes more common in boys or girls?
> Boys

1410. Patients with Perthes commonly present with what complaints?
> Painless limp and knee pain

1411. On exam, what motion is typically lost?
> Abduction and internal rotation

1412. What is the association between age at diagnosis and prognosis?
> Age <6 years old at diagnosis is associated with better outcomes

1413. If bilateral, should lesions be in the same stage of disease?
> No, if symmetric think Multiple Epiphyseal Dysplasia (MED) or thyroid disorders
> 15% of Perthes is bilateral, but will not be in the same stage of disease

Slipped Capital Femoral Epiphysis (SCFE)

1414. What is SCFE?
> Slippage of the proximal femoral metaphysis relative to the epiphysis

1415. How do you determine clinically if a SCFE is stable or unstable?
> Loder Classification
  - Stable: Able to bear weight (even with crutches)
  - Unstable: Unable to bear weight

1416. What is the classification for SCFE slip severity?

Pediatrics

> Southwick Classification – the difference between femoral epiphyseal diaphyseal angles of both hips
>   - Mild: <30°
>   - Moderate: 30-50°
>   - Severe: >50°

1417. What is the epiphyseal diaphyseal angle?
> Angle between a line drawn perpendicular to the proximal femoral epiphysis and a line drawn along the femoral diaphysis

1418. What constitutes an acute SCFE?
> Symptoms for <3 weeks

1419. What is the direction of slippage?
> Metaphysis slips anteriorly and externally rotates, epiphysis stays within the acetabulum

1420. Through what zone of the physis do SCFEs occur?
> Hypertrophic zone

1421. What types of patients are at a higher risk for SCFE?
> Obese adolescent boys

1422. What percentage of patients have bilateral involvement?
> 25%

1423. What radiographs should be obtained for a stable slips?
> AP pelvis, frog leg lateral

1424. What type of lateral radiograph should be obtained if a SCFE is unstable?
> Shoot through lateral

- Frog leg position may exacerbate slip and should be avoided

1425. What is Klein's line?
    - A line drawn along the superior femoral neck should intersect the epiphysis in a normal hip on an AP radiograph

1426. What are the indications for an endocrine work up?
    - Atypical SCFE: <50th percentile for weight, <10 years old, and valgus slips

1427. What is the most common cause of non-idiopathic SCFE?
    - Hypothyroidism

1428. Why do patients with SCFE commonly complain of medial knee pain?
    - Referred pain from the anterior branch of the obturator nerve

1429. What unique physical exam finding is seen in a patient with a SCFE?
    - Obligatory external rotation of the hip with passive flexion

1430. How are SCFEs most commonly treated?
    - In situ fixation with cannulated screws

1431. How many threads should cross the physis?
    - 5 threads, less is associated with slip progression

1432. How do you confirm that the screw is not in the hip joint?
    - Approach-Withdraw technique: Hip range of motion on fluoroscopy

Pediatrics

1433. During the treatment of an unstable SCFE with in situ screw fixation your attending slides an instrument along the femoral neck, why?
> Capsulotomy
  - Decompression of the capsule theoretically decreases the risk of AVN

1434. When is prophylactic fixation of the contralateral hip considered?
> Patients with endocrine abnormalities, age <10 years old, and contralateral hip pain

Transient Synovitis vs Septic Arthritis

1435. What are the Kocher criteria?
> Set of values that help distinguish between transient synovitis and septic arthritis
  - Inability to bear weight
  - Serum WBC >12k
  - ESR >40
  - Temperature >101.3°F

1436. What is the probability of septic arthritis with 4, 3, 2, 1, and 0 criteria present?
> 4: >99%
> 3: 93%
> 2: 40%
> 1: 3%
> 0: <1%

1437. What additional lab value, can help make this distinction?
> CRP>20 mg/l

Pediatrics

1438. What is the diagnostic study of choice to rule out a septic hip?
> Ultrasound with aspiration if an effusion is present

1439. What position is the hip generally held in if septic?
> Flexion, Abduction, External Rotation (FABER)
  - This position allows for the greatest volume within the hip capsule

1440. How is transient synovitis treated?
> Anti-inflammatory medications

Femur

1441. What is the classification for pediatric femoral neck fractures?
> Delbet Classification
  - Type I: Transphyseal
  - Type II: Transcervical
  - Type III: Cervicotrochanteric/Basicervical
  - Type IV: Intertrochanteric

1442. What are the different treatment modalities for fixing femoral shaft fractures?
> Pavlik harness
> Spica cast (immediate or delayed)
> Flexible intramedullary nails
> Rigid intramedullary nail
> ORIF
> Submuscular plate
> External fixator

Pediatrics

1443. What is the treatment of choice for patients with femoral shaft fractures who are <6 months of age?
> Pavlik harness

1444. What are the two most common treatment modalities for femoral shaft fractures in patients who are 6 months to 5 years of age?
> Spica casting, flexible nails

1445. What are the contraindications for using flexible nails?
> Length unstable fractures, weight >50 kg (110 pounds), age >11 years old

1446. What is the recommended flexible nail size compared to canal diameter?
> Goal is 80% canal fill, 40% from each nail
> - Note: Nails should be the same size

1447. What starting point should be used for rigid intramedullary nails in pediatric patients?
> Lateral trochanteric starting point

1448. Why is the lateral trochanteric starting point recommended for rigid intramedullary use in pediatric patients?
> Increased AVN risk with more medial starting points due to injury to the medial femoral circumflex artery

1449. What is the reported rate of AVN with the piriformis, greater trochanter, and lateral entry starting points?
> Piriformis: 2%
> Greater trochanter: 1.4%
> Lateral entry: 0%

Leg Length Discrepancy (LLD)

1450. Generally, half of the final leg length occurs at what age in boys and girls?
   - Girls: 3 years old
   - Boys: 4 years old

1451. What radiographs should be obtained when evaluating a patient with LLD?
   - Full length, standing radiographs of the bilateral lower extremities

1452. What is the first line of treatment for patients with LLD of <2cm?
   - Shoe lift

1453. What are the two treatment categories for patients with LLD of 2-5cm?
   - Shortening the long side – epiphysiodesis
   - Lengthening the short side – distraction osteogenesis

1454. What two categories of implants can be used for limb lengthening?
   - Circular external fixator, intramedullary nail

1455. How fast are you able to lengthen an extremity during the distraction phase?
   - Up to 1mm/day

1456. What is the name given to the new bone that is formed?
   - Regenerate

Blount's Disease

1457. What is Blount's disease?

> Abnormal development of the proximal posteromedial tibial physis

1458. What coronal plane deformity is seen with Blount's disease?
    > Genu varum
1459. What are the two types of Blount's disease?
    > Infantile (early onset): 0-3 years old, more common, more severe
    > Adolescent (late onset): >10 years old
1460. What radiographic finding is seen with early onset Blount's disease?
    > Medial metaphyseal beaking
1461. What is Drennan's angle and how do you measure it?
    > Metaphyseal-diaphyseal angle: Angle created by a line perpendicular to the long axis of the tibia and another line connecting the metaphyseal beaks
1462. What Drennan's angle is considered pathologic?
    > >16°
1463. What physical exam finding is indicative of a pathologic process rather than physiologic genu varum?
    > Varus thrust with ambulation indicating lateral collateral ligament insufficiency
1464. What deformity may be seen in the distal femur in patients with Blount's?
    > Compensatory valgus

Tibia

1465. What fracture in kids is the equivalent to an ACL rupture in an adult?

Pediatrics

- ➢ Tibial spine fracture

1466. What is the classification for tibial spine fractures?
- ➢ Meyers and McKeever Classification
  - Type I: Nondisplaced
  - Type II: Anterior displacement, intact posterior hinge
  - Type III: Completely displaced
  - Type IV: Displaced and comminuted

1467. What two structures commonly block the reduction of a tibial spine fracture?
- ➢ Anterior horn of the medial meniscus or the intermeniscal ligament

1468. What are the classifications for tibial tubercle fractures?
- ➢ Ogden Classification
  - Type I: Anterior fracture through tubercle apophysis
  - Type II: Through apophysis extending between apophysis and epiphysis
  - Type III: Through apophysis and epiphysis
  - Type IV: Extends across the entire proximal tibial physis
  - Type V: Periosteal sleeve avulsion
- ➢ Pandya Classification
  - Type A: Tubercle Youth – ossified tip fracture
  - Type B: Physeal – epiphysis and tibial tubercle fracture as a unit off of the metaphysis; extra-articular
  - Type C: Intra-articular

- Type D: Tubercle Teen – fracture to the distal aspect of tubercle (closed physis)

1469. What devastating complication can occur following tibial tubercle fractures?
> Compartment syndrome

1470. Which Pandya type has the highest risk of compartment syndrome?
> Type B

1471. What artery is thought to be responsible for compartment syndrome following tibial tubercle fractures?
> Recurrent anterior tibial artery

1472. What deformity results from growth arrest of the tibial tubercle?
> Recurvatum

1473. What is Cozen's phenomenon?
> Development of a late valgus deformity following proximal tibial metaphyseal fracture

1474. What types of tibial bowing are present in the pediatric population?
> Anterolateral, anteromedial, and posteromedial tibial bowing

1475. Based on x-ray, how do you name tibial bowing?
> Named for the apex of the bow

1476. What conditions/characteristics are associated with each type of tibial bowing?
> Anterolateral ("Bad Bowing"): Neurofibromatosis Type I, pseudoarthrosis
> Anteromedial: Fibular hemimelia

Pediatrics

> Posteromedial ("Good Bowing"): Physiologic, calcaneovalgus foot, leg length discrepancy
>   - Remember: **P**ostero**M**edial = **P**robably **M**ild

Ankle

1477. What is the classification system for pediatric ankle fractures?
    > Dias and Tachdjian Classification
    >   - Supination Inversion: SH I fibula, SH IV tibia
    >   - Supination Plantarflexion: SH II posterior tibia
    >   - Supination-External Rotation: Metaphyseal tibia and fibula
    >   - Pronation/Eversion-External Rotation: Suprasyndesmotic fibula fracture, SH II tibia

1478. What is a Tillaux fracture?
    > SH III of the anterolateral distal tibia

1479. What ligamentous structure is attached to the Tillaux fragment?
    > AITFL (Anterior Inferior Tibiofibular Ligament)

1480. Why does the Tillaux fracture happen in this anatomic location?
    > Last portion of the distal tibial physis to close
    >   - Remember: Closes central to medial to lateral

1481. What is the reduction maneuver for a Tillaux fragment?
    > Plantarflexion and internal rotation

1482. What is a triplane fracture?
    > Complex SH IV injury with fractures in three planes (axial, coronal and sagittal)

Pediatrics

1483. With a triplane fracture, what fracture patterns are seen on the AP and lateral x-rays?
> AP: SH III (sagittal plane)
> Lateral: SH II (coronal plane)

1484. What type of mechanism typically leads to Triplane and Tillaux fractures?
> External rotation force

Foot

1485. What deformities contribute to clubfoot?
> **C**avus (midfoot)
> **A**dductus (forefoot)
> **V**arus (hindfoot)
> **E**quinus (hindfoot)
> - Remember: "**CAVE**"

1486. What is the treatment of choice for clubfeet?
> Ponseti casting

1487. With Ponseti casting, what is the order of deformity correction?
> Cavus → Adductus → Varus → Equinus

1488. The foot is rotated laterally around what anatomic structure during Ponseti casting?
> Talus

1489. When clubfoot recurs, which deformity occurs first?
> Equinus

1490. What position is the foot in with a congenital vertical talus (CVT)?
> Extreme forefoot dorsiflexion with a rigid rocker bottom foot

1491. What radiograph is used to evaluate for CVT?
> Maximal plantarflexion view

1492. How do you distinguish CVT from an oblique talus?
> Oblique talus: Talonavicular joint reduces on the maximal plantarflexion radiograph

1493. What are the two most common anatomic types of tarsal coalitions?
> Calcaneonavicular (most common)
> Talocalcaneal

1494. What radiographic sign is seen with a calcaneonavicular coalition?
> Anteaters sign

1495. What radiographic sign is seen with a talocalcaneal coalition?
> "C" sign

1496. Tarsal coalitions decrease motion at which joint?
> Subtalar joint

1497. What injury do patients with tarsal coalitions commonly have?
> Recurrent ankle sprains due to the inability to accommodate uneven surfaces

1498. What is Kohler's disease?
> AVN of the tarsal navicular

1499. What is Sever's disease?
> Calcaneal apophysitis

1500. What is Iselin's disease?
> Apophysitis of the tuberosity of the proximal 5th metatarsal

Question Index

The Basic – Pg. 1
<u>X-rays</u>
Upper Extremity 1-15
Pelvis 16-29
Lower Extremity 30-44
<u>Infections</u> 45-74
<u>Compartment Syndrome</u> 75-94
<u>General Knowledge</u>
AO/OTA Classification 95-98
Nonunions 99-102
Closed Fractures 103
Open Fractures 104-114
Osteoporosis 115-124
Cartilage 125-128
Bone Formation 129-133
Principles/Properties 134-150

Shoulder Girdle – Pg. 25
<u>General Anatomy</u> 151-191
<u>Trauma</u>
Clavicle 192-202
Acromioclavicular (AC) Joint 203
Scapula 204-205
Proximal Humerus 206-216
Shoulder Dislocation 217-226
<u>Sports</u>
Rotator Cuff 227-241
Instability & Labrum 242-263
Proximal Biceps 264-267
Adhesive Capsulitis 268-276
<u>Adult Reconstruction</u>
Hemiarthroplasty 277-280
Arthroplasty 281-291
Reverse Arthroplasty 292-297

Arm – Pg. 49
<u>General Anatomy</u> 298-307
<u>Trauma</u>
Humerus 308-323

Elbow – Pg. 55
<u>General Anatomy</u> 324-359
<u>Trauma</u>
Capitellum & Trochlea 360-361
Proximal Ulna 362-367
Proximal Radius 368-373
<u>Sports</u>
Elbow Instability 374-382
Epicondylitis 383-388
Distal Biceps 389-395

Forearm & Wrist – Pg. 67
<u>General Anatomy</u> 396-421
<u>Trauma</u>
Forearm 422-426
Wrist 427-449

Hand – Pg. 77
<u>General Anatomy</u> 450-509
<u>Hand Conditions</u>
Carpal Tunnel Syndrome 510-516
Scaphoid 517-534
Lunate 535-540
Metacarpal 541-550
Thumb 551-561
Phalanx 562-569
Trigger Finger 570-572
Flexor Tendons 573-582
Extensor Tendons 583-589
CMC Arthritis 590-592

Spine – Pg. 97
<u>General Anatomy</u> 593-617
<u>Trauma</u>
Vertebral Fractures 618-621
Spinal Cord Injuries 622-635
<u>Spinal Conditions</u>
Cervical Myelopathy 636-639
Ankylosing Spondylitis 640-643
DISH 644-646

Pelvis – Pg. 107
<u>General Anatomy</u> 647-663
<u>Trauma</u>
Pelvic Ring 664-680

Hip – Pg. 113
<u>General Anatomy</u> 681-701
<u>Trauma</u>
Acetabulum 702-714
Hip Dislocations 715-723
Femoral Head & Neck 724-737
Intertrochanteric Fxs 738-743
Subtrochanteric Fxs 744-748
<u>Sports</u>
FAI 749-755
Snapping Hip 756-758
<u>Adult Reconstruction</u>
Total Hip Arthroplasty 759-788

Question Index

Femur – Pg. 133
<u>General Anatomy</u> 789-797
<u>Trauma</u>
Femoral Shaft 798-820
Distal Femur 821-827

Knee – Pg. 139
<u>General Anatomy</u> 828-867
<u>Trauma</u>
Patella 868-873
Knee Dislocations 874-883
Tibial Plateau 884-896
<u>Sports</u>
ACL 897-924
MCL/LCL 925-934
Meniscus Injuries 935-943
Discoid Meniscus 944-949
Patella 950-969
<u>Adult Reconstruction</u>
TKA 970-1015
UKA 1016-1020

Leg – Pg. 167
<u>General Anatomy</u> 1021-1032
<u>Trauma</u>
Tibial Shaft 1033-1043

Foot & Ankle – Pg. 173
<u>General Anatomy</u> 1044-1106
<u>Trauma</u>
Pilon 1107-1116
Ankle 1117-1138
Talus 1139-1145
Subtalar Dislocations 1146-1150
Calcaneus 1151-1166
Lisfranc 1167-1177
5th Metatarsal 1178-1183

<u>Foot & Ankle Conditions</u>
Achilles tendon 1184-1193
Peroneal Tendons 1194-1197
Post. Tibial Tendon 1198-1204
Hallux Valgus 1205-1217
Hallux Rigidus 1218-1223
Cavovarus Foot 1224-1241
Freiberg's Disease 1242-1245
Lesser Toes 1246-1251

Pediatrics – Pg. 201
<u>General Anatomy</u> 1252-1266
<u>The Basics</u>
Physis 1267-1275
Joint Hypermobility 1276-1277
Lower Ext. Alignment 1278-1283
Cerebral Palsy 1284-1286
<u>Upper Extremity</u>
Little Leaguer's Shoulder 1287-1289
Supracondylar Humerus 1290-1307
Elbow 1308-1322
Forearm & Wrist 1323-1329
Hand 1330-1343
Upper Ext. Syndromes 1344-1347
<u>Spine</u>
Scoliosis 1348-1366
Kyphosis 1367-1370
Spondy 1371-1380
<u>Lower Extremity</u>
DDH 1381-1406
Legg-Calve-Perthes 1407-1413
SCFE 1414-1434
Synovitis vs Septic Hip 1435-1440
Femur 1441-1449
Leg Length Discrepancy 1450-1456
Blount's Disease 1457-1464
Tibia 1465-1476
Ankle 1477-1484
Foot 1485-1500

Notes

Notes

Notes

Notes

Notes

Notes

Notes